LIVING WITH

Alex Gazzola is an author, journalist and writing who has written widely on health, nutrition and lifestyle *Living with Food Intolerance* is his second book.

Overcoming Common Problems Series

Selected titles

A full list of titles is available from Sheldon Press,
36 Causton Street, London SW1P 4ST and on our website at
www.sheldonpress.co.uk

Overcoming Common Problems

Living with Food Intolerance

Alex Gazzola

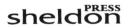

First published in Great Britain in 2005
Sheldon Press
36 Causton Street
London SW1P 4ST

Copyright © Alex Gazzola 2005

British Library Cataloguing-in-Publication Data

A catalogue record for this book is available from the British Library

ISBN 0–85969–939–0

1 3 5 7 9 10 8 6 4 2

Typeset by Deltatype Limited, Birkenhead, Merseyside
Printed in Great Britain by
Ashford Colour Press Ltd

Contents

Acknowledgements

Enormous gratitude to the many sufferers of food intolerance who volunteered their experiences and tips for this book. And to Dr Sarah Brewer, Dr Damien Downing, Anne-Marie Holdsworth, Dr Catti Moss, and especially to Christine Baker and Muriel Simmons – each of whose expertise illuminated my understanding of the subject.

Introduction

What is food to one man, may be fierce poison to another.
Lucretius, 75AD

Who shall decide, when doctors disagree,
and soundest casuists doubt, like you and me?
Alexander Pope (1688–1744)

To eat is human, to digest divine.
Mark Twain (1835–1910)

The food sensitivity problem

IS YOUR FOOD HARMING YOU?

Barely a week goes by without a newspaper or magazine carrying this kind of worrying headline somewhere. It is attention grabbing – but alarmist.

That food can be detrimental to our health is currently a matter of widespread concern. New fad diet plans, food scares such as BSE, pesticide residues in our fruit and vegetables – such topics are regularly subjected to media scrutiny and speculation, much of it welcomed by an increasingly knowledgeable public with an apparently insatiable appetite to learn more.

The resulting commercialization of nutritional advice has created an ever-expanding army of self-appointed dietary gurus, some of whom dispense sweeping, often conflicting and ill-reasoned recommendations to sometimes vulnerable and baffled consumers: 'Don't ever eat wheat! Beware red meat! Avoid mixing your carbs and proteins!'

But what is often forgotten, or ignored, is the good food does us. Food nourishes us, providing our bodies with the building blocks they need to grow, replenish and stay healthy. It fuels us, allowing us to work and play. It brings us immense sensory pleasure and satisfaction. It is central to our family rituals, social occasions and religious festivals. Children kindle friendships through sharing bags of sweets; lovers seduce one another over oysters and chocolate strawberries; parents bond intimately with their babies and children at feeding time.

In more ways than one, food gives us life.

Yet, we know that individuals can be affected not by food per se, but perhaps one or several specific kinds of food, ingredients in foods or constituents of foods. Possibly the most notorious example of this is a classical food allergy, caused by an inappropriate and dramatic action towards a food of the immune system – the system of cells responsible for keeping the body free from infection.

The culprit is usually a protein – for instance, a specific protein in peanuts – and the reaction itself is characterized by the rapid onset of a number of sometimes frightening symptoms, such as tingling in the mouth, a skin rash, wheezing or asthma, diarrhoea and vomiting. In hypersensitive individuals, such adverse responses can be triggered by exposure to even an exquisitely minute particle of the offending food.

In extreme cases, an allergic reaction can result in anaphylaxis, where the blood pressure plummets, the mouth and throat (and perhaps other tissues) swell dangerously, breathing becomes increasingly laboured and the body collapses into unconsciousness (called anaphylactic shock). Unless medical attention is sought at once, or a dose of the hormone adrenalin is promptly administered intramuscularly, it can be fatal within minutes.

Mercifully, anaphylaxis is rare – but food allergy in general is less so. According to the British Nutrition Foundation, food allergies affect 0.2–0.5% of adults. But Allergy UK – a charitable organization offering support and advice to sufferers of all food and chemical sensitivities – puts the figure as high as 2%, while a report entitled *Allergy: The Unmet Need*, published by the Royal College of Physicians in 2003, states 'over 3% of the population' are now affected by true food allergy.

What is not in dispute, however, is that numbers are rising steadily. The cause is uncertain.

Food intolerance

But not all unwelcome reactions to foods are as dramatic or potentially serious as allergic ones. In the last decade or so, a different kind of food sensitivity has taken increasing prominence in the public's consciousness.

Food intolerance is the subject of this book, and its symptoms are far less specific than those of food allergy. Typically, these are often associated with other conditions or illnesses and can take a while to materialize – up to three days after consumption – often making diagnosis difficult. Among them are a runny nose, headaches, abdominal pains, bloating, diarrhoea, constant tiredness, restlessness and an inability to concentrate – symptoms which aren't necessarily dangerous or harmful, but which sufferers could certainly do without. They can be regular, or they can come and go sporadically; they can steadily worsen over time, remain consistent in their severity, or – more rarely improve of their own accord.

As will become clear, this sort of idiosyncratic unpredictability is typical of food intolerance. It is far from being a thoroughly understood science.

Controversy surrounds it too. With research in the field sadly lacking, estimates for numbers of sufferers in the UK differ wildly, from 2% to 60% of the adult population – and these are statistics sourced from various health bodies, medical experts and nutritionists. As is so often the case with such disparate views, the truth probably lies somewhere in between – but meanwhile, it is confusing to those seeking relief from their ill-health.

Even the causes of food intolerance are not entirely agreed upon. Some suspect psychological factors – that people convince themselves that they are, for instance, intolerant to gluten, whereas in fact their symptoms are caused by stress, distress or other factors quite distinct from their daily bread. Others implicate the heavy reliance on wheat and dairy products in our modern western diet of ready meals and fast food, not to mention the preservatives and other additives routinely thrown in to prolong shelf-life and enhance appearance. Are symptoms of food intolerance the body's way of fighting back? Nature signalling that we should broaden our diets and thereby expose ourselves to a wider range of wholesome foods and the nutrients associated with them?

While there aren't as many clear-cut answers as we would like when it comes to food intolerance, this book aims to separate fact from fiction, from an independent point of view. It will define and explain what food intolerance is and is not, what the causes are or might be, and which symptoms may be indicative of an intolerance.

If you suspect you may be a sufferer, later chapters will explain how you can best obtain a diagnosis, and how, once the one or more culprits have been identified, you can then manage, live with and in many cases resolve your food intolerance.

Lastly, we will give you some sound advice on how to prevent recurrences or new intolerances developing in future.

1
Allergies and intolerances: the differences

Many people mistakenly use the terms 'allergy' and 'intolerance' interchangeably. It would be unfair to blame them. Instead, we should probably view this as an unfortunate consequence of the disagreement that rumbles on among members of the nutritional, medical and allergological fields over precise meanings and usage – a confusion which appears to have filtered down through the media to the lay public.

Hence, it is impossible to give undisputed definitions of food allergy and food intolerance. If you consult other reports or titles on adverse reactions to food – particularly those from other English-speaking countries – you may find slight variations to those used here. The two that follow are by no means definitive or unanimously agreed upon, but they will apply throughout this book.

A *food allergy* is a prompt, inappropriate and potentially dangerous response of the immune system to a constituent of a food which to most other people is perfectly harmless. The substance responsible is called an allergen, which is normally a protein – for instance, one found in peanuts, tree nuts or fish. Typical signs include rashes, wheezing, vomiting and angioedema (swelling of the lips, mouth and throat).

A *food intolerance* is a delayed, unpleasant, but never directly life-threatening response to one or more foods which may or may not involve the immune system to some extent. It is characterized by a far broader catalogue of symptoms than that of food allergy, and it can affect different people in very different ways. Among its manifestations are gastric and digestive disturbances, skin problems, fluid retention, lethargy, insomnia, headaches and any number of other generic complaints.

Because the diagnosis, management, treatment and prognosis of the two conditions differ so greatly, it is important to have a clear understanding of allergies before we consider intolerances in greater depth. To that end, let us look more closely at both kinds of food sensitivity, beginning with allergies.

What triggers a food allergy?

An allergic reaction to a food occurs when the body's immune system encounters a substance it mistakenly considers to be a threat

1

– that is, an allergen which has passed into the body, usually via oral ingestion or through the skin. In particularly sensitive individuals, merely the smell of a culprit food can elicit a reaction – the allergen entering through the nasal lining or lungs.

In order for the immune system to deem the protein dangerous enough to warrant such drastic action, it must previously have been exposed to it and subsequently have developed 'sensitization' to it. Initial exposure to an allergen can happen when very young. A child can be fed the allergen-containing food directly, consume it via the mother's breastmilk, or even receive it as an embryo through the placental bloodstream. The process of sensitization is essentially an overreaction of the immune system to an innocuous 'invader'. Anxious to confer protection on the body, the immune system responds to a new and suspect allergenic protein by manufacturing chemicals called antibodies to tackle it.

The antibodies involved in classical food allergies are called Immunoglobulin E – or IgE for short. Once formed, the IgE antibodies attach themselves to immune cells called mast cells. In the main, mast cells are found where the body is most vulnerable to invasion from microbes – such as the nose and lung.

When an individual comes into contact with an allergen to which sensitization has been established, the allergen and its corresponding IgE antibody bind. This binding causes the host mast cell to be activated and release inflammatory substances, such as the chemical histamine, in what can be described an immunological 'call to arms'.

Problems occur when the sheer volume of released chemicals cause unwanted changes in the body. These include swelling, rashes, diarrhoea and vomiting – all designed to flush out the 'invader'. Unfortunately for the patient, these reactions can be distressing, debilitating and, at worst, life-threatening.

It is unclear why some people are more susceptible than others to allergy. Hereditary malfunction of the immune system – known as atopy – is one probable cause. Sensitization as an infant, before the immune system is mature enough to deal properly with the proteins typically associated with allergy, is a second.

Sufferers need to keep antihistamine medication close at hand to counter the effects of an unexpected allergenic exposure. Those susceptible to anaphylactic responses are strongly urged to always carry an Epi-Pen, with which they can self-administer a dose of potentially life-saving adrenaline should they inadvertently come into contact with a food to which they are severely allergic.

It is imperative that you see your doctor if you suspect you have an allergy. Doctors are well versed in IgE-mediated reactions, and are ideally positioned to properly advise you. Support groups such as Allergy UK can also help.

Food intolerance

Reactions to foods not caused by an IgE immune response are much more prevalent, and most can be classified as food intolerance. Many are not well-understood or even accepted by the medical orthodoxy, and there is no typical scenario to offer as standard, as each individual demonstrates an entirely unique repertoire of symptoms which can vary in time of onset, intensity, duration and order of presentation.

Which foods cause intolerance?

Any person can develop a food intolerance, and just about any food can be responsible for it. However, the most common problem foods tend to be those consumed regularly and/or in relatively large quantities. These are:

- wheat and related grains, and foods containing them, such as breads, pastas, cereals, cakes and biscuits;
- dairy products, such as milk and cheese;
- eggs, either the white, the yolk or both;
- yeast-containing foods, such as breads, yeast extract, vinegars, beers and wines;
- sugars and sweets;
- some meats; soya and soya products;
- citrus fruits, especially oranges;
- alcoholic drinks;
- coffee, tea and chocolate;
- processed foods, rich in additives.

All these pervade the average UK diet. In the USA, intolerance to corn – a common component of the American diet – is more widespread. Intolerance to rice – rare in the West – is often reported in south and east Asia.

What are the symptoms?

This is a difficult question to answer – and the source of much controversy. Some delayed reactions – diarrhoea, migraine and bloating, for instance – to certain foods are accepted. More unusual symptoms reported or claimed – such as impotence, incontinence and restless leg syndrome – are wisely viewed more cautiously.

What *is* known is that food intolerance can exacerbate existing symptoms as well as incite new ones. These symptoms can affect almost any part of the body, and many are digestive and/or inflammatory manifestations. Below is a list of those which are wholly or mostly accepted as genuine possible responses to certain foods in susceptible individuals – although, of course, all have alternative causes.

Gastro-intestinal symptoms

Loss of appetite, halitosis (foul breath), nausea, vomiting, ulcers, indigestion, stomach pain; and also abdominal pain, cramps, bloating or distension, borborygmi ('tummy gurgles'), flatulence, diarrhoea, constipation – sometimes collectively dubbed or diagnosed as irritable bowel syndrome (IBS).

Respiratory and cardiac symptoms

Wheezing, coughing, asthma, shortness of breath, heart arrhythmia (irregular heartbeat or palpitations).

Symptoms of the skin

Eczema, dermatitis, itching, urticaria (rashes/hives), angioedema, acne, psoriasis.

Symptoms of the ear, nose, throat and eyes

Rhinitis (nasal inflammation), post-nasal drip, sinusitis and blocked nose, otitis media ('glue ear'), itchy ear, eye irritation.

Muscular or physical symptoms

Myalgia (muscular pain and stiffness), arthritic pain, tiredness, lethargy, weakness, weight fluctuation, oedema (fluid retention).

Symptoms of the head and mind

Headache, migraine, insomnia, dizziness, mental slowness.

Emotional symptoms

Indifference, mood swings, depression, restlessness, panic attacks, emotional eating, antisocial behaviour.

Immunological symptoms

Low or compromised immunity, difficulty in fighting off infection.

All can begin almost imperceptibly and worsen steadily over the years, until they become chronic conditions. Alternatively, they can be triggered by a particular viral illness, incidence of food poisoning or period of intense stress.

Symptoms can flare up, calm down, come and go erratically. A particular reaction to a particular food one day, may become an entirely different reaction to the same food another day, may become no reaction whatsoever on yet another day. Quite often, the symptoms are bothersome but mild; rarely, they're strong.

Some individuals 'collect' intolerance reactions over the period of their illness, beginning with gastric symptoms and progressing to further symptoms affecting the skin, for example. By the time they seek treatment, a desperate few have amassed a portfolio of conditions which threaten to overwhelm their ability to function normally from day to day – what has started as a sensitivity to one food, may have become a sensitivity to several.

Sufferers of chronic food intolerance can find their immune systems compromised by continual ill-health, weakening their ability to fight off disease, leaving them open to further medical complications (including other intolerances). This cyclical pattern of progressively worsening health can cause desperate misery for those affected so adversely.

Further complicating matters is the fact that most of the symptoms of food intolerance are 'masked' – in other words, they are often associated with other, unrelated conditions or diseases. This makes diagnosis difficult. We will be returning to symptoms in Chapter 3.

Causes of food intolerance

Unlike food allergy, which has one clear-cut mechanism, there are several known or possible causes of food intolerance, some of which may operate collaboratively to bring about symptoms. The most important are considered below.

Enzyme deficiencies

Enzymes are substances the body manufactures to bring about vital chemical reactions.

Digestive enzymes, for instance, break down the constituents of the food we eat into smaller units the body is able to absorb and utilize. If the body lacks or does not produce enough of a particular digestive enzyme, undigested food particles can upset the body in numerous ways.

Detoxification enzymes, on the other hand, help break down natural toxins found in everyday foods into harmless compounds which can then be excreted from the body. In their absence, the toxins may linger and also cause unpleasant side-effects.

IgG antibodies

Immunoglobulin G (IgG) is a class of antibody thought by many working in the field to be responsible for a substantial share of food intolerances. Advocates of the IgG theory blame 'leaky gut syndrome' (LGS) – a condition in which an individual's gut wall becomes abnormally permeable.

Where there is a leaky gut, it is thought that indigestible or undigested food molecules are able to pass through the gut wall and into the bloodstream, where they're set upon by the body's immune system. But rather than being attacked by IgE antibodies as in classical food allergies, they are targeted by IgG antibodies, which tend to provoke delayed, rather than immediate, responses in some individuals.

Auto-immune responses

By far the most common example here is coeliac disease – a lifelong disorder caused by a unique form of intolerance to gluten, a protein found in wheat, rye, barley and some other grains.

In coeliac sufferers, gluten is believed to precipitate an auto-immune – or self-attacking – reaction which 'eats' away at the food-absorbing cells of the small intestine, in turn preventing the efficient uptake of nutrients. Symptoms vary, but often include exhaustion, bloating, flatulence, diarrhoea, malnutrition and weight loss. The disease is managed by following a gluten-free diet – usually effective in restoring sufferers to good health. Coeliac disease is further considered in Chapter 6.

Reactions to non-nutrients

These can occur in response to pharmacologically active compounds in foods – for example caffeine in coffee, which may cause symptoms such as tachycardia (rapid heartbeat) and insomnia. Other naturally occurring chemicals can, in sensitive individuals or when consumed in unusually large quantities, provoke toxic reactions – as can some additives. These include the natural toxin solanine (in potatoes), the flavour enhancer monosodium glutamate (MSG) and the colouring tartrazine.

These reactions can be attributed to a lack of a particular detoxifying enzyme or to the direct action of the offending chemical on the body. Reactions to non-nutrients are considered in Chapters 10 and 11.

Psychogenic mechanisms

Sometimes referred to as somatization disorders, these are responses precipitated by the mind and not through an automatic physiological mechanism in the body.

For instance, someone convinced that dairy products are causing their unpleasant symptoms may well experience those symptoms when consuming a cup of milky tea. However, if unknown to the sufferer the milk is disguised or hidden in another food or dish – say, in an omelette – no such adverse reactions will occur. Psychogenic reactions are considered in Chapter 12.

Idiosyncratic reactions

These are responses which at present resist classification or definition, and may well be caused by elements of human biology which are poorly understood or yet to be discovered. Doctors sometimes refer to them as 'idiopathic' – prosaically, this means 'cause unknown'.

Food sensitivity: a definition

Because the line dividing food intolerance and food allergy is a little blurred, the term food sensitivity is sometimes used as an umbrella – or 'catch all' – term.

A *food sensitivity* can be defined as an unwelcome and reproducible physiological reaction to food. (Note that this definition excludes psychogenic reactions.) But for our purposes, the distinctions between food allergy and food intolerance are important, and worth re-emphasizing. With that in mind, Table 1 summarizes the major differences between the two.

Table 1: Differences between food allergies and food intolerances

Food Allergies	Food Intolerances
Produce acute, distinctive symptoms within seconds or minutes	Produce masked symptoms, usually within between half an hour and three days
Mediated by IgE antibodies	Mediated either by non-IgE or non-immunological mechanisms
Can be life-threatening	Not directly life-threatening
Not dose dependent: even a tiny quantity of the culprit food can effect a reaction	Dose dependent: a substantial portion of the culprit food is usually required to provoke a reaction
Can be triggered through oral contact or ingestion, or cutaneous or respiratory contact	Can only be triggered through ingestion
The culprit food is avoided and not craved	The culprit food is regularly eaten in quantity and often craved
Usually, a sufferer reacts only to one or two foods	Often, a sufferer will react to several foods

2
Digestion, immunity and leaky gut

Food intolerance tends to manifest itself in otherwise healthy individuals when normal digestive processes either work inefficiently or incompletely, are somehow hindered, or do not take place at all. This in turn can lead to unwanted reactions and the unpleasant symptoms associated with them.

Anybody's digestive system can malfunction. To see how and why, we first need to consider how a healthy digestive system should ideally work when food is introduced into the body.

What is digestion?

Most food is of no use to the body in the form in which we consume it. It first needs to be broken down into smaller constituents which the body can then absorb and reassemble to suit its own needs – for instance, to build new cells or to nourish and fuel existing ones. This process is called *digestion*.

It occurs in the digestive tract (or alimentary canal): the tube which starts at your mouth, takes in the oesophagus (gullet), stomach, small and large intestines, and ends – approximately nine or ten metres later – at your bottom.

The catalysts which help dismantle the food into simpler molecules are called digestive enzymes. Many of the enzymes and chemicals required for digestion are produced in the salivary glands, the liver, the gall bladder and the pancreas – vital organs which together with the digestive tract constitute the entire digestive system (see figure 1).

Which foods does the body need?
Proteins, carbohydrates and fats ('macronutrients'), vitamins and minerals ('micronutrients'), fibre and water are all required.

Proteins are provided mostly by meats, fish, eggs, grains, nuts and dairy products. The body breaks proteins down into amino acids before it can assimilate them and use them to build muscle, skin and other new cells.

Complex carbohydrates (starches) are found in breads, pasta, whole-grains, pulses, fruits and vegetables while *simple carbohydrates* (sugars) are found in dairy products, fruit, vegetables and refined

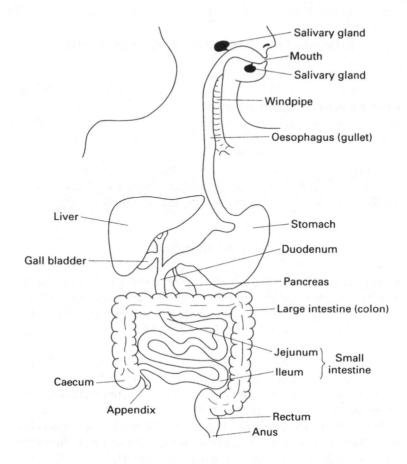

Figure 1: The digestive system

sweet products. Unless already in their simplest state, all dietary carbohydrates must be reduced to their constituent molecular units before the body can efficiently exploit them as fuel sources.

Fats are found in meats, fish, eggs, nuts, butter and oils. The body breaks down fat into glycerol and fatty acids. They are important for healthy nerves, hormones, hair, skin and as a storable energy source.

Vitamins and *minerals* are present in virtually all foods, and are required in modest amounts for a diversity of complex biological processes, from the formation of bone to the regulation of the cardiovascular system.

Fibre, strictly a form of indigestible carbohydrate found in all plant foods, provides bulk and keeps the digestive system clean, fit and working efficiently.

Water is arguably the most essential nutrient of all, one without which we would die within days. Every essential chemical process in the body occurs in its presence.

What happens in digestion?

This is best considered stage by stage.

The mouth

Food is introduced into the body through the mouth, whose primary digestive task is to thoroughly chew and lubricate food with saliva, making it easier to swallow. Saliva also contains amylase, an enzyme which begins the process of starch digestion.

The oesophagus (gullet)

This is the flexible, muscular tube, lined with a mucous membrane, which leads from the mouth to the stomach. The oesophagus moves food down into the stomach by peristalsis – a wavelike massaging and pushing which is a trait of the entire digestive tract.

The stomach

This is a muscular J-shaped bag, located under the rib cage. It has a number of functions: to receive and store food and liquid; to churn up food until it becomes a sludgy semi-liquid called chyme; to secrete through its mucous membranes hydrochloric acid (to begin the breakdown of protein and sterilize food), the enzyme pepsin (to further advance the digestion of protein) and a little lipase (an enzyme which digests fats); to absorb water and any alcohol; to feed chyme into the duodenum in conveniently spaced and sized 'portions'.

The small intestine

At around six or seven randomly coiled metres, the term 'small intestine' may appear a misnomer, but the name is a reference to its narrow width. It consists of three parts – the duodenum, the jejunum and the ileum – and it is here that most digestion and absorption of food takes place.

When food from the stomach arrives, the short *duodenum* receives bile from the liver and gall bladder, and enzymes and sodium bicarbonate from the pancreas. Bile emulsifies any fats present in preparation for digestion. The pancreatic enzymes include amylase (to digest carbohydrates), lipase (to digest fats, assisted by bile) and trypsin (to digest protein), while the bicarbonate partially neutralizes the acidic chyme. Minerals, simple sugars, vitamins and digested fats are absorbed into the body in the duodenum.

From the duodenum, food is pushed into the *jejunum* – about three metres long – whose mucous membranes also secrete an assortment of enzymes – called brush border enzymes – to further assist digestion. The jejunal wall absorbs fats and amino acids, as well as simple sugars and vitamins.

Further vigorous peristalsis moves food on into the *ileum* – roughly four metres in length – which absorbs water-soluble vitamins, amino acids, cholesterol and recyclable bile salts.

Most of the small intestine's lining is characterized by an elaborate, undulating network of small finger-like projections and 'micro-projections' called villi and microvilli, respectively. This serves to dramatically increase the surface area available for the absorption of digested foods through the cells of the mucosal gut membranes.

These membranes also secrete an important non-inflammatory antibody called secretory Immunoglobulin A (sIgA), which defends against microbes and binds to any reactive food molecules. This process ensures foreign substances and undigested proteins are made too chemically large to cross the gut wall, so they are mainly excluded – unlike digested nutrients of small molecular size, which are usually efficiently absorbed.

The large intestine or colon

The three principal parts of the colon are the ascending colon, the transverse colon and the descending colon. The colon's main task is to receive the remnants of the digestive process from the small intestine and to manufacture stool from them, which can then be passed out of the body. It also recycles water, reabsorbing it into the system along with some simple nutrients such as mineral salts.

Like the small intestine, the large intestine contains bacteria, but on a much bigger scale – at any time, each of us has about a kilo or more in our colons. Most are beneficial, forming a vital part of the immune system; some are disease-causing. Benevolant bacteria – commonly called probiotics – keep any pathogenic bacteria and natural yeasts in the gut at bay, and manufacture absorbable vitamins B and K. Furthermore, they digest fibre, producing fatty acids which aid colonic function.

As the developing stool progresses up, across and down the large intestine via contractions, and assisted by secretions of mucus from the gut wall, it gradually changes from liquid to solid as fluid absorption takes place. By the time it reaches the lower descending colon, it is properly formed.

The rectum

Stool from the descending colon collects in the rectum. When a sufficient quantity is present, a message is sent to the brain to signify the rectum is ready to be emptied.

The anus

This is the opening to the end of the digestive tract where formed stool leaves the body, rounding off the process of digestion.

What can go wrong?

It is only to be expected in such a sophisticated system of delicate interconnecting organs that digestive functioning can dip below optimal levels, sometimes because of illness, stress or natural ageing. Of most concern in relation to causes of food intolerance are: enzyme deficiencies, leaky gut syndrome (LGS), immune responses to food, intestinal bacteria and yeasts, and an overworked liver.

Enzyme deficiencies

Two possibilities present themselves. In the first, a particular enzyme which specializes in digesting a specific constituent of food can either be entirely absent from the body or in permanently short supply. Such a deficiency can be hereditary. For example, in the case of a deficiency of lactase – the enzyme needed to digest the dairy sugar lactose – undigested lactose passes through the small intestine and into the colon, where it is met by bacteria that feast on it, fermenting it, causing flatulence, abdominal pain and frothy diarrhoea.

Alternatively, normal enzyme production can, under certain conditions, be impeded, insufficient or suppressed. The reasons for this may include: our tendency of washing down meals with beverages and juices, which may have a diluting effect on digestive enzymes; the overconsumption of processed foods, leading to a low intake of natural plant enzymes; and inflammation or damage to sites in the small intestine which secrete enzymes, hampering their output.

Food molecules which remain in their undigested state – because of an enzyme problem or otherwise – can be absorbed through the gut wall and into the bloodstream where, unrecognised by the immune system as food, they may be targeted by it. This is believed by some to be the key mechanism involved in establishing an IgG-mediated food intolerance (see below).

13

Detoxification enzyme deficiencies can also have negative effects. If the multi-tasking liver is burdened with other metabolic processes, it may be unable to produce enough enzymes needed to cope with a sudden workload – such as an evening's drinking. Similarly, exposure to environmental or other toxins may overtax the liver to such an extent that its digestive duties may be neglected.

Leaky gut and the immune response

All our guts are leaky – but some are more leaky than others; and the leakier the gut, the more likely larger undigested molecules are to pass through it.

Factors which may contribute to a leakier gut include: medicines (including antibiotics), anti-inflammatory painkillers (ibuprofen, aspirin), the Pill, recreational drugs; alcohol, tobacco and caffeine; refined sugars, processed foods and food additives; spicy foods (chilli, strong curry); localized allergic inflammatory reaction to an undigested protein; chronic stress; environmental toxins; food poisoning/gastroenteritis; bacterial imbalance and parasitic yeast overgrowth (see below).

Undigested food molecules can challenge the small intestine. Normally, any with reactive capacity are targeted by sIgA, reducing the likelihood of their penetrating the gut wall. However, if sIgA levels are low – because of stress, poor nutrition, localized inflammation or hereditary deficiency, for instance – fewer of these proteins become deactivated, leaving more free to permeate the mucous membranes.

It ought to be stressed that these food molecules penetrate the gut walls of the healthiest individuals. Ideally, the immune system binds many of them to non-inflammatory IgA antibodies in the blood, after which they are efficiently dealt with by immune cells.

But, in what is a disputed area, some researchers believe that in certain circumstances more inflammatory IgG antibodies rather than gentle IgA antibodies are formed to food. Why this may happen is unclear.

Once IgGs form to a food, the theory is that the body effectively becomes sensitized to it. When the food molecules penetrate the gut wall again in their undigested state, tailor-made IgG antibodies bind to them and trigger a range of reactions, many of which are inflammatory and which strain the body's defences. This may be why many people feel tired after dining on a meal rich in the foods to which they are unwittingly intolerant: the hard-at-work immune system is sapping all the body's available energy, leaving it exhausted.

A further consequence of a leaky gut is the extra demands it places on the liver, which may then become overstrained, possibly compromising its detoxification mechanisms.

Gut flora

Present in the intestines of every human are billions of bacteria and yeasts, of several hundred species, collectively known as the gut flora.
Bacteria For our purposes, we can apply a three-way categorization: healthy – or probiotic – bacteria; pathogenic – or disease-causing – bacteria; commensal bacteria (neither here nor there).

Fortunately, in a healthy intestine the good bacteria stay on top of the bad by maintaining an acidic environment which is 'antisocial' to the pathogenic group.

But sometimes the balance of power is upset. When disease-causing microbes get a chance to multiply, a condition called dysbiosis results. Possible contributory factors to dysbiosis include: heavy or repeated use of broad-spectrum antibiotics; chronic stress; poor nutrition (processed foods, refined sugars) and fad dieting; overeating; slow intestinal transit time/sluggish bowels; severe illness (such as diabetes); multiple pregnancies; chemical exposure.

In dysbiosis, pathogenic bacteria can damage the intestinal mucous membrane. Again, that means a leakier gut.
Yeasts Alongside gut bacteria live yeasts. One controversial idea is that overpopulation of these fungi can ultimately lead to symptoms of food intolerance. Many apportion blame directly on a particular yeast – candida albicans.

Overgrowth of candida and the toxins it produces can provoke gut inflammation and damage brush border enzymes, possibly leading to – you've guessed it – LGS, but also to mineral malabsorption, an overloaded immune system and liver and, not implausibly therefore, food intolerance.

Aside from the typical undesirable symptoms of dysbiosis – abdominal pain or distension, flatulence – other reactions sometimes pinned on candida dysbiosis include poor mental functioning, headache and irritability.

So what causes food intolerance?

All or any of the conditions described above may be triggering or contributing to symptoms of food intolerance. Often they co-exist, because one particular malfunction or disorder can directly cause one or more of the others – and indeed be caused by them.

3

Symptoms and signs

Symptoms are your body's way of registering its discontent. Those associated with food intolerance are many and varied. Some can provide pointed clues to their sources. Others can baffle the most informed of specialists.

What follows is a look at each of the principal symptoms typically associated with delayed reactions to food. The list cannot be exhaustive. Because each of us is characterized by a unique lifestyle, medical history, and biological and physical make-up, food sensitivities in different individuals will manifest themselves in an abundance of ways.

Neither should it be used as a diagnostic tool. Self-diagnosis of lactose intolerance to frequent diarrhoea and abdominal pain may well be accurate, but can you afford to risk missing a graver possibility?

Remember that even those of glowing health suffer occasionally from the symptoms listed. The causes are often mundane and nothing to do with food sensitivity. You can easily rule out some of these yourself. For instance, if you jog daily, you can in all confidence eliminate 'lack of exercise' as a source of your sporadic constipation. With others, you will of course need your doctor's help. If after relevant tests he, or a specialist, can find nothing else wrong with you, then food intolerance should be considered.

Bear in mind too that symptoms of food intolerance usually present in number rather than individually, range in intensity from mild to highly unpleasant, and are generally delayed (although some chemical intolerances, for instance, can appear within half an hour or less and feel severe). Often they are chronic or long-standing symptoms, which can present sporadically.

A final note of caution: a mild and regularly felt discomfort in your tummy may well reveal itself to be a long-undetected delayed reaction to wheat fibre; but the out-of-nowhere onset of apocalyptic abdominal pain has nothing to do with food intolerance, and everything to do with an intestinal blockage, twisted bowel or other medical emergency.

So please use what follows wisely.

Abdominal pain/cramps

Often precursors to diarrhoea. Common in irritable bowel syndrome (IBS).

Food intolerance?

Very possibly. Common in coeliac disease, lactose intolerance and chemical intolerances, among others.

Other digestive causes

Low calcium intake; trapped wind; peptic ulcer; gastro-intestinal cancers; diverticulitis; pancreatitis; appendicitis; inflammatory bowel diseases (IBDs) such as Crohn's disease or ulcerative colitis; gut obstruction or strangulated hernia.

Unrelated causes

Nervous tension; pre-menstrual syndrome (PMS), endometriosis; peritonitis.

Angioedema

see *Urticaria and angioedema*

Anorexia

The loss of appetite, in which hunger is absent (the illness characterized by a distorted perception of one's body, extreme weight loss and a morbid fear of weight gain is, strictly speaking, anorexia nervosa). Anorexia may present with an absence of saliva.

Food intolerance?

Uncommon, but possible.

Other digestive causes

Zinc deficiency; gastritis, gastroenteritis or intestinal inflammation; appendicitis; Crohn's disease; stomach cancer.

Unrelated causes

Anxiety, stress and depression; extreme illness.

Arthritis and arthralgia

Joint inflammation and joint pain, respectively.

Food intolerance?

Sometimes a symptom in coeliac disease. Commonly implicated in

IgG-mediated intolerances, via the mechanism of immune complex deposition in joints. Typical offending foods include gluten grains, dairy, pork and other meats. Corn and sunflower oils, and the nightshade vegetables (tomatoes, potatoes, aubergines, peppers) may be problematic too.

Other digestive causes
Gut dysbiosis and LGS; gastroenteritis; inflammatory bowel disease (IBD).

Unrelated causes
Stress; physical injury; environmental pollution; viral infections; immune disorders.

Asthma and wheezing

Difficulty breathing due to temporarily narrowed airways; may be accompanied by coughing or tightness in the chest. Those affected may be atopically predisposed to asthma, and a number of factors can precipitate attacks or worsen symptoms.

Food intolerance?
Possibly, if symptoms are intermittent. Wheat and dairy often blamed for childhood wheezing, as are eggs, nuts, fish and chocolate – but whether this is an intolerant or allergic reaction isn't always clear. Chemical intolerances – especially of sulphites – are commonly implicated.

Other digestive causes
Poor diet/excess junk food; diet high in margarines/saturated vegetable fats and low in olive oils/oily fish; bloating in stomach; obesity.

Unrelated causes
Exposure to pollution, tobacco smoke, feather bedding, chlorine swimming baths or cold air; over-exercising (aerobic); true allergy (to pollen, animal dander, spores etc.); viral or bacterial infection; panic or shock, excitement or laughter – all can bring on symptoms.

Bad breath

see *Halitosis*

Bloating

Or abdominal distension, common in IBS sufferers.

Food intolerance?

Possibly coeliac disease or a carbohydrate intolerance, in tandem with other symptoms.

Other digestive causes

Consumption of gassy drinks, rich fatty meals and gas-producing foods (see Flatulence); rushed eating; gut dysbiosis; IBD.

Unrelated causes

Stress; pre-menstrual syndrome.

Blocked nose

see *Sinusitis*

Borborygmi

The Latin name for bowel noises, or tummy rumbles or gurgles, often caused by intestinal contractions 'stirring' up semi-liquid contents. Not usually troublesome in themselves.

Food intolerance?

Possibly, along with other symptoms. Common in the carbohydrate intolerances.

Other digestive causes

Hunger; Crohn's disease; intestinal obstruction.

Unrelated causes

Fear or anxiety.

Constipation

Very infrequent opening of bowels, inability to pass a motion, or having to strain on the loo.

Food intolerance?

Unlikely, unless intermittent with diarrhoea, which could imply IBS. With bloating, it can occasionally signify a wheat or wheat fibre intolerance.

Other digestive causes

Low-fibre diet, irregular meals, overreliance on refined or junk food, low fluid intake, abrupt change in diet; gut dysbiosis; diabetes; diverticulitis; painkillers, iron tablets, medicinal drugs.

Unrelated causes

Ignoring the call of nature; lack of exercise; change of living routine; stress, tension and anxiety; depression; anorexia nervosa; pregnancy or menopause; laxative abuse; thyroid problems; post-anaesthesia.

Cramps

see *Abdominal pain/cramps*

Craving

The urge to consume a certain food; if not met, any number of unpleasant psychological and physiological symptoms can result (palpitations, irritability).

Food intolerance?

Regular feature of many food intolerances. Wheat and milk cravings are strong signs of intolerance, particularly in children. One intriguing theory is that consumption of some intolerance-causing foods triggers the release of 'feelgood' hormonal changes in the body, to which individuals become 'addicted'.

Other digestive causes

Mineral deficiency; dysbiosis (especially a sugar/yeast craving); hypoglycaemia (sugar craving).

Unrelated causes

Anaemia (meat craving); pregnancy; food addiction; veganism (protein craving).

Depression

see *Emotional disturbance*

Dermatitis (atopic)

see *Eczema/atopic dermatitis*

Diarrhoea

Watery or runny stools; often the main feature of IBS.

Food intolerance?

A common symptom, implicated in: coeliac disease, lactose intolerance and transient lactose intolerance (for instance, during infection), fat intolerance due to lipase or bile deficiencies (resulting in fatty diarrhoea), intolerance to some fruits or fruit sugars, and some chemical intolerances.

Other digestive causes

Niacin deficiency; sudden change in diet; food poisoning or contaminated water (often when abroad); gut dysbiosis and LGS; diverticulitis; IBD; colon cancer.

Unrelated causes

Stress and emotional tension; sustained physical exertion (e.g. marathon running); laxative abuse; antibiotics; poor hygiene.

Dizziness

A sense of spinning, movement, light-headedness or shaky balance.

Food intolerance?

Possible, but uncommon. Perhaps an intolerance to a food additive.

Other digestive causes

Food poisoning.

Unrelated causes

Anxiety and worry; low blood pressure, hypoglycaemia; diabetes; viral illness; labyrinthitis, Ménière's syndrome; allergy; certain medication; toxic pollution in the home; pregnancy; anaemia.

Dyspepsia

see *Indigestion*

Eczema/atopic dermatitis

A skin condition typified by itchy, dry, scaly and sometimes cracked, red and inflamed skin.

Food intolerance?

As with asthma, the distinction between allergy and intolerance is often unclear with regard to eczema. Children are especially vulnerable. Dairy intolerance often presents with eczema on the knees. Other culprit foods identified by a number of studies include wheat, eggs, fish, soya, tomatoes and peanuts. A form of dermatitis, called dermatitis herpetiformis, is linked to gluten intolerance.

Other digestive causes

Candida dysbiosis and LGS; deficiency in zinc or essential fatty acids.

Unrelated causes

Allergy; bath soaps, shower gels and moisturizers; detergent traces on washed clothing.

Emotional disturbance

Including, but not limited to, mood swings, depression, restlessness, hyperactivity (in children), as well as indifference, irritability, panic attacks, emotional eating, antisocial behaviour, aggression . . .

Food intolerance?

Very possibly. Linked to some enzyme deficiencies and chemical intolerances.

Other digestive causes

Yeast dysbiosis and LGS; poor dietary choices and fad dieting (especially low-carbohydrate diets or low-fat diets); alcohol abuse; caffeine withdrawal; folic acid deficiency.

Unrelated causes

Drug or nicotine abuse or withdrawal; bereavement; social rejection; serious illness; bed confinement; life transition; post-natal depression; seasonal affective disorder (SAD); anaemia; natural hormonal fluctuations (in adolescence, or pregnancy).

Exhaustion

see *Tiredness*

Fibromyalgia (FM)

Often widespread pain and stiffness in the muscles and tendons.

Food intolerance?

Possibly implies a lack of digestive enzymes.

Other digestive causes

LGS; liver malfunction; low calcium intake.

Unrelated causes

Influenza; next-day response to physical exertion; lack of exercise; stress and nervous tension; failure to relax; insomnia.

Flatulence

Gas in the intestine, released via the rectum. It is normal to break wind around twenty times daily.

Food intolerance?

Excessive flatulence can imply an intolerance to wheat fibre, lactose or other sugars.

Other digestive causes

Gut dysbiosis; consumption of gas-producing foods, including: beans, onions, cabbages, sprouts, cauliflower, onions and garlic; gum chewing.

Unrelated causes

Certain antibiotics.

Fluid retention

see *Oedema*

Glue ear

see *Otitis media*

Halitosis

Commonly known as 'bad breath'. Often, the sufferer is oblivious to the problem.

Food intolerance?

Occasionally. It is often a symptom of gut dysbiosis, and a 'sub-symptom' of constipation. In the latter case, slowly transitting waste matter can ferment excessively in the gut and create foul, noxious gases then absorbed through the walls of the sluggish colon and into the bloodstream, later excreted in the breath.

Other digestive causes

Consumption of garlic, onions, spices, and other strong-flavoured foods; low hydrochloric acid levels in the stomach.

Unrelated causes

Dental or gum disease; poor oral hygiene; liver or kidney disease; undiagnosed diabetes.

Headache and migraine

Headache becomes migraine when it becomes incapacitating.

Food intolerance?

Regularly implicated, with numerous possible villains. Chocolate (especially dark), red wine and strong cheeses are the classic migraine-causing foods because of their high amine content, but wheat, dairy, egg, citrus fruits, sugars and some additives are also suspected.

Other digestive causes

Dehydration (common in ordinary headaches); gut dysbiosis and LGS; fasting and fad dieting; cold food (typically ice cream); caffeine withdrawal ('weekend headache syndrome'); alcohol abuse.

Unrelated causes

Too little/much sleep; bright lights, loud music or other external stimuli; hypoglycaemia; stress and overwork; stiff neck; abrupt meteorological changes; PMS; environmental pollution; overreliance on painkillers.

Heart arrhythmia (irregular heartbeat)

Poundings of the heart are termed palpitations; accelerated heartbeat is tachycardia.

Food intolerance?

Possibly a chemical intolerance, such as to caffeine or the amines.

Other digestive causes

Excessive alcohol or caffeine intake.

Unrelated causes

Excitement, fear or anger; excessive smoking; certain medication; thyroid illness; problems with heart muscles or valves, or general heart disease.

Heartburn

see *Indigestion*

Hives

see *Urticaria*

Hyperactivity

see *Emotional disturbance*

Immune malfunction

As typified by low or compromised immunity to common viruses, or slowness in fighting off an infection.

Food intolerance?

Common in IgG-mediated intolerances or coeliac disease.

Other digestive causes

Gut dysbiosis and LGS; malnutrition, typically a low intake of fruits and vegetables and a high-fat or highly processed or sugary diet.

Unrelated causes

Excessive stress or feeling 'run down'; lack of exercise; ageing; atopy; serious illness.

Indigestion

A partial misnomer, in that it does not necessarily imply compromised or non-digestion (generally termed *mal*digestion). More often, it is characterized by bloating or discomfort in the upper abdomen, possibly heartburn, and belching. Sometimes called dyspepsia.

Food intolerance?

Sometimes, if present with other symptoms. Wheat, coffee and (unfiltered) tap water can precipitate indigestion, while coffee, tea, mint and mint tea, chocolate, milk and tomatoes can underlie heartburn.

Other digestive causes

Eating too much, too quickly, when standing up, irregularly, late at night or when stressed, tense or excited; very hot/cold food; lying down after a meal; consuming excess alcohol or fruit juices with food; spicy, acidic or fatty food; fizzy drinks; gallstones; peptic ulcer; hiatus hernia.

Unrelated causes

Lack of exercise, obesity; smoking; pregnancy; anxiety or stress; steroids, non-steroidal anti-inflammatory drugs (NSAIDs) and antibiotics.

Insomnia

The inability to fall or remain asleep.

Food intolerance?

Possibly, if an enzyme deficiency has left undigested food in the system. Dairy intolerance in particular can cause insomnia.

Other digestive causes

A heavy evening meal and/or eating late; caffeine and alcohol; heartburn.

Unrelated causes

Lack of exercise; heavy sleep the previous night or a long lie-in that morning; smoking and other stimulant drugs; stress and nerves; jet lag; snoring partner; disturbed night-time breathing (sleep apnoea); poor quality mattress; weak bladder or prostate problems.

Itchiness

Skin irritation relieved short-term by scratching.

Food intolerance?

Possibly, as per eczema and urticaria. Some – especially children – who are intolerant to citrus fruits will suffer itchy symptoms.

Other digestive causes

Parasitic dysbiosis (anal or vulval itching).

Unrelated causes

Perfumes and toiletries; synthetic fabrics or washing liquid residues on clothing; scabies; insect bites; jaundice; psychological mechanisms (you may start to itch merely by reading this).

Joint pain

see *Arthritis*

Lethargy

see *Tiredness*

Loss of appetite

see *Anorexia*

Migraine

see *Headache and migraine*

Mood swings

see *Emotional disturbance*

Nausea and vomiting

Gastric disquiet or the sensation of being about to expel food from the stomach via the mouth, and the uncontrollable act of doing so.

Food intolerance?

Very possibly, common in several intolerances.

Other digestive causes

Hunger (nausea only); fatty food; too much tea or coffee; peptic ulcer, gastritis, alcohol abuse, oesophagitis (gullet inflammation due to hot, spicy or strong food); magnesium deficiency; appendicitis; Crohn's disease.

Unrelated causes

Nicotine abuse; distress or shock; viral infections or fever; pregnancy; true allergy; somatization disorder; head injury; inner ear infection; travel motion.

Oedema

More prosaically, fluid retention and associated puffiness and swelling, typically on the lower legs, hands, abdomen and chest.

Food intolerance?

Occasionally.

Other digestive causes

High salt/low fluid intake; low protein diet; yeast dysbiosis; alternate binge eating/starvation dieting.

Unrelated causes

Prolonged inactivity; liver disease or kidney disease; chronic lung disease; PMS; poor circulation; steroid use; pregnancy.

Otitis media ('Glue ear')

Bacterial inflammation of the middle ear, common in children.

Food intolerance?

Regularly reported. Usual suspects are wheat, milk, soya, peanuts and eggs.

Unrelated causes

Bacterial infection of the nose and throat, spreading to the ear; smoking or smoke exposure.

Pain (abdominal)

see *Abdominal pain/cramps*

Pain (joints)

see *Arthritis and arthralgia*

Pain (muscular)

see *Fibromyalgia (FM)*

Palpitations

see *Heart arrhythmia*

Psoriasis

A genetically inherited disposition to thick, scaly reddened patches of skin, especially on elbows and arms, knees, lower legs, feet, back and scalp.

Food intolerance?

Possibly. Some have linked psoriasis to enzyme-deficient protein intolerance, and to consumption of the nightshade vegetables.

Other digestive causes

Yeast dysbiosis and LGS; low hydrochloric acid in the stomach (affecting protein digestion); poor liver function; high consumption of alcohol, meat or sunflower and corn oils.

Unrelated causes

Skin creams, stress, viral infections, sunburn and cold weather can all trigger an attack.

Rashes

see *Urticaria*

Restlessness

see *Emotional disturbance*

Rhinitis, rhinorrhoea and sinusitis

Respectively, inflammation of the nose, a runny nose and inflammation of the mucous membranes – leading to sneezing, blockage, discomfort and itchiness, for instance.

Food intolerance?

Possibly, but more common in allergy. Chemical intolerances can cause nasal symptoms. Dairy produce is popularly blamed for encouraging mucus production, but conclusive evidence is lacking.

Other digestive causes

Hot spicy food can cause severe short-lived rhinorrhoea.

Unrelated causes

Allergy (especially hay fever, or dust mite and animal dander allergies); colds and influenza; smoke or fumes; artificial smells such as synthetic perfumes; nasal polyps or growths; obstructions; cold air; medicinal drugs; recreational drugs; pregnancy; thyroid disease.

Stiffness

see *Fibromyalgia (FM)*

Swelling

see *Oedema* and *Urticaria and angioedema*

Tiredness

Physical tiredness may present with weakness, lethargy, exhaustion; mental tiredness is characterized by inability to concentrate, mental sluggishness and sleepiness. 'Tired all the time' (TATT) is a common complaint.

Food intolerance?
Very possibly, especially if in the hour or two after a meal. Wheat and dairy often blamed.

Other digestive causes
Gut dysbiosis and LGS; hypoglycaemia; incipient diabetes; diet rich in sugar, fat and refined foods; alcohol consumption; iron, folic acid, vitamin B12 or vitamin C deficiencies.

Unrelated causes
Depression; anaemia; late pregnancy and breastfeeding; thyroid problems; recent illness or serious disease; keeping unusual hours; chronic fatigue syndrome/ME; anorexia nervosa or low body weight; obesity; stress and personal problems; disturbed sleep.

Ulcers (oral or peptic)

Mouth ulcers we all get from time to time, but recurrent ulcers are a problem. Peptic ulcers in the stomach (gastric ulcers) show themselves as a burning pain across the chest; those in the duodenum (duodenal ulcers) as pain in the middle of the abdomen, around two hours after eating.

Food intolerance?

Uncommon, but chronic mouth ulcers are a symptom of coeliac disease. Dairy intolerance another possibility.

Other digestive causes

High alcohol consumption; IBD (mouth ulcer); iron or vitamin B deficiencies (mouth ulcer); infection with helicobacter pylori bacterium (gastric ulcer); high intake of refined carbohydrates, pickled food and possibly dairy as it is acid producing (gastric ulcer).

Unrelated causes

Smoking; dentures, poor dental hygiene, sharp dental edges (mouth ulcers); stress (gastric ulcers).

Urticaria and angioedema

Urticaria – also known as hives or nettle rash – is an itchy pink or red rash caused by fluid leakage in the capillaries below the skin's surface. Angioedema is a deeper, more swollen form of urticaria, in which the blood vessels leak fluid, leading to puffiness, typically around the lips, mouth, throat and eyelids. The two often co-occur.

Food intolerance?

A common reaction. Often, an intolerance to food additives or toxins are to blame. Fruit or its juices can cause transient urticaria; alcohol can exacerbate it.

Other digestive causes

LGS.

Unrelated causes

Allergy; latex sensitivity; some medicines, such as aspirins or NSAIDs, and antibiotics (particularly penicillins); sun exposure; aerobic exercise; some forms of auto-immune disease; pressure on the skin.

Vomiting

see *Nausea and vomiting*

Weakness

see *Tiredness*

Weight problems

Loss or fluctuation of weight; also, the inability to *gain* weight. (Obesity or being overweight is *not* a recognized consequence of food sensitivity.)

Food intolerance?

A common chronic symptom of coeliac disease or other malabsorptive condition.

Other digestive causes

Yeast dysbiosis; exaggerated caffeine consumption; IBD; pancreatitis.

Unrelated causes

Anorexia nervosa; heavy smoking; anaemia; diabetes; thyroid problems.

Wheezing

see *Asthma*

Wind

see *Flatulence*

4

Tests and diagnoses

You may by now have a hunch about whether your symptoms might be related to food and, if so, which foods may be responsible. Naturally, you want a firm diagnosis to allow you to take action. So how to go about it?

First, it is important you keep an open mind. Doctors and dietitians often remark that patients come to them with fixed beliefs about their condition, which can hinder progress. Second, be aware that it might not be easy to obtain a diagnosis. In contrast, a classical allergy is relatively uncomplicated to confirm through recognized methods such as skin prick testing (SPT) or blood tests for IgE antibodies. Doctors feel 'comfortable' with such tests. They produce visible results and fairly reliable indications. When tests for forms of intolerance are available, results may not always be so clear-cut.

In addition, some members of the medical profession are sceptical of certain forms of intolerance and about numbers of sufferers. There may be numerous reasons for this, including scant coverage of food allergy and intolerance on the undergraduate medical syllabus, and scarcity of solid clinical research.

Further compounding matters is the paucity of allergy and intolerance provision within the NHS. Ideally, some forms of intolerance should be managed by a trained allergist. However, in the UK there are only a handful of full-time and part-time allergy clinics staffed by such specialists, with some supplementary part-time services offered by consultants in other specialties. But their geographical distribution is unevenly concentrated in London and the south east, leaving the Celtic nations and the north and south west of England woefully underserved.

But even those lucky enough to win on the postcode lottery can't always get a referral to a specialist clinic, or for that matter to a state registered dietitian. Furthermore, waiting lists can be long for both. For any number of reasons, patients can get disillusioned, with two common results – they self-diagnose, or they turn to alternative practitioners.

Self-diagnosis

A typical scenario reported by doctors and dietitians is this. A patient – often, but not always, a woman under forty – may suffer symptoms after eating, for instance, a pizza. She may attribute those reactions to wheat and cheese, especially after reading an unbalanced article blasting the 'evils' of both foods. She will remove them from her diet. Should she then suffer a reaction to, say, rice, she may eliminate that too. And so on. Until, eventually, she's eating a sparse diet which is starving her of vitamins, minerals and proteins, and ends up at her healthcare provider feeling worse than she did before.

Worryingly, it has also become increasingly fashionable to declare oneself 'intolerant' to validate embarking on a restricted diet of some sort – typically a 'cleansing' one. Newspaper headlines such as 'I lost twenty pounds by giving up wheat, dairy and eggs!' printed alongside a picture of an impossibly svelte celebrity do not help.

Do bear in mind that restricting on a whim the food you eat can leave you undernourished, and many so-called detox diets can have the same effect if you follow them indefinitely.

Admittedly, these regimes *can* quickly clear up symptoms in some. The foods typically vetoed – breads, dairy, eggs, red meats, sugar, coffee – are among those most commonly blamed for food intolerance. The more you subtract from your diet, the more likely your particular culprit or culprits will be among them.

Yet this is *not* a recommendation. First, if you remove dozens of foods and your symptoms improve, you will be no closer to discovering which, if any, food adversely affects you. Second, your diet could be nutritionally incomplete, and you may end up feeling considerably worse, not better. Third, such diets can send you spiralling towards a permanently unhealthy relationship with food, and all the unwanted consequences that may bring.

If you have mild symptoms, Allergy UK suggests keeping a food diary (see page 36) for a fortnight, recording everything you eat, any responses, and their severity. Once complete, look back to see whether there are any obvious associations between a particular food and particular reactions.

Then, if one food is suspected, try cutting it out for a month, replacing it with a substitute that ensures your nutrient intake is not compromised (for example, fortified soya milk for milk, rice for potatoes, or pears for apples). If you improve, continue for up to three months, and then reintroduce the food gradually into your diet, but only once every four days initially.

Ideally, though, Allergy UK concedes that it is always preferable you work with a doctor and dietitian. This is vital when you suspect more than one food to be culpable, when your symptoms are more alarming, or when you're concerned you may have coeliac disease, for instance. It is imperative in *all* cases involving children – under no circumstances should you restrict a child's diet without medical approval and supervision.

Alternative practitioners

Just as the perennial fashion for dieting has spawned a thriving industry of 'nutritionists' touting questionable weight-loss regimens, so the increase in food sensitivity and the dearth of healthcare provision have produced fringe therapists promising first to diagnose you, then provide you with miraculous cures. All for a handsome fee, of course.

Please beware. Absurd proclamations are regularly made and – sadly – believed. Watch out for the depressingly common use of pseudo-scientific terminology such as 'negative force fields' and 'blocked energy paths', or the assertion to cure your sensitivity through hypnosis or auto-suggestion. Some private practitioners, clinics and high-street health stores offer suspect and unvalidated diagnostic tests, some of which we will consider in Chapter 5. Most complementary therapies – designed to 'complement' not replace conventional treatments – are harmless, and may deliver limited benefits – although you should always be wary of glowing and subjective endorsements often served up in print media.

The possible danger comes with alternative therapies, marketed to the public as substitutes for conventional diagnoses and treatments. When fringe practitioners stray into territory which orthodox medicine rightly holds should be the strict preserve of dietitians, and begin imposing potentially unsafe food restrictions based on unreliable test results, patients can suffer badly.

Should you see your doctor?

If your responses are mild, occasional, or you are not overly bothered by them, then you may not need to see your doctor. Everybody endures infrequent bouts of indigestion, excess wind and erratic bowel movements, for instance. This is normal.

You might want to implement a sensible lifestyle change based on an idea from the previous chapter, or if relevant, you could try the simple elimination suggested earlier. If you're seeing your doctor on an unrelated matter, take the opportunity to discuss your symptoms.

If your complaints are abdominal, the following home beetroot test may help you make a more informed choice. It offers an approximation of your intestinal transit period – the time food takes to travel from mouth to bottom.

Dine on a meal rich in beetroots. Three will suffice. They should stain your stools, something you'll notice when you wipe. Calculate the time between consumption and the first purple stool. Do this several times, leaving a week between tests, to calculate an average.

Under twelve hours may signify malabsorption, possibly indicating an underlying problem such as an enzyme deficiency, coeliac disease, a pancreatic disorder, low bile production, high stomach acidity, gut dysbiosis or Crohn's disease. See your doctor.

Eighteen to thirty-six hours is generally considered ideal, but there is some disagreement among specialists, so don't be unduly alarmed if you fall a little outside these parameters.

Over forty-eight hours, and especially over seventy-two hours, suggests constipation and the wide range of problems associated with it. Try drinking more water, eating more fruits and vegetables and taking more exercise for several weeks, then retest yourself. Ongoing constipation should be referred to your doctor.

Note. This test is merely intended as a guide. It cannot diagnose or rule out any condition or intolerance; it is not suitable for those for whom dark stools are a regular occurrence (in which case, see your doctor urgently) or who are sensitive to oxalates (see page 82).

If you are worried, or you have new, severe or persistent symptoms which are troubling you and perhaps worsening, or have any doubts at all about your health, it's important you make an appointment specifically – if only to give yourself an objective second opinion or to eliminate the more sinister, albeit remote, possibilities.

The food diary

Keeping a food and symptom diary for two weeks prior to your appointment is a great help. From it, you may be able to identify an obvious connection between a dietary component and a reaction. If you can't, your doctor (or a dietitian) might.

Aim to do it properly for it to be of value. Every food, every activity and every symptom should be recorded – as you go along. The memory is fallible; if you write entries at the end of the day you'll omit key details.

A typical page might look like this:

Monday 25 July 2005

Time	Food and drink	Activity	Symptoms
8am	two slices wholemeal toast, a little butter and two dessert-spoons of low-sugar apricot jam; two cups black coffee	watching TV	
9am			normal bowel movement; no straining or pain
10am	200ml tap water	twenty-minute jog	
11am	apple and glass of milk		
12am			constant hunger pangs

Here are some tips on keeping a useful diary:

- use a light, portable notebook;
- devote a page for each day;
- if you are mostly at home, keep the diary in the kitchen so it is handy when you prepare food;
- write clearly so your healthcare professional won't struggle to read it;
- do not alter your diet or routine – the point is to identify whether anything you eat or do normally is causing problems;
- be specific – note portion sizes, the form in which you eat a food (raw, fried, boiled, etc.), the contents of a prepared food (cut out the ingredients label and stick it in your diary, if it helps), and even the order in which you eat foods at a sitting;
- include easily forgettable items such as chewing gum or breath fresheners, any medication or painkillers, and glasses of water (tap, mineral, still, filtered or sparkling);
- record the duration and severity of symptoms: use a scale of 1 (mild) to 5 (severe).

The consultation

Prepare yourself for the questions your doctor might ask. These include: When and how did your symptoms begin? What do you think triggers them? Have you taken any medication for them? Are they exacerbated by stress? Do you suffer from allergies, such as hay fever? Is there a history of intolerance in your family?

You will of course need to discuss your diet, lifestyle and symptoms in detail – this is where any home testing or your diary can help.

Tests

Your doctor will examine and test you. Among the possible procedures are: weight measurement; examination of the ears, nose and throat; basic heart and lung checks; pulse and blood pressure measurement; palpation, where the doctor feels your abdomen; urine test, possibly to check for sugar, a diabetes indicator, or protein, a sign of possible kidney disease; rectal examination.

There are other tests, some of which your doctor may be able to administer. Others may be attended to by a consultant at a clinic or hospital.

Blood tests

Tests can confirm lactose intolerance when taken before and after you have been given a lactose drink – a diagnosis being arrived at if blood glucose levels fail to rise substantially.

If coeliac disease is a possibility, a test called the tissue transglutaminase test may be carried out (see *Endoscopy*, page 40).

With extreme gastro-intestinal symptoms, your doctor may want to look for blood markers suggestive of IBD.

A blood test may also be used to test for raised cholesterol, anaemia, immune antibodies, impaired liver or kidney function, and pancreatitis.

Breath tests

The urea breath test may be used to detect helicobacter pylori bacteria in the stomach, implicated in gastric ulcers. It involves swallowing a substance which the bacteria break down into gases then detectable in the breath.

A hydrogen breath test can confirm lactose intolerance. After drinking some milk, your breath is tested for hydrogen at regular intervals. A positive result confirms the intolerance.

Pulmonary tests

If you are experiencing wheezing, a peak flow meter test may be arranged to test for asthma. The meter is a gadget which measures the speed at which you exhale air. You may be loaned one and asked to keep a diary of readings.

The spirometry test is performed to confirm asthma. The spirometer measures the rate and volume of air exhaled.

Stool tests

A faecal occult blood test (FOB) identifies traces of blood in your stools. Consecutive positive results imply a bleeding bowel. Further tests will be needed.

A stool sample may be tested for parasites, viruses or bacteria.

Specialist referrals

Your doctor might refer you to a dietitian (see Chapter 5), or send you to a specialist for further tests or for the management and treatment of a confirmed diagnosis. For instance, for wheezing you may be referred to a lung specialist, and for urticaria or eczema to a dermatologist. If the conditions co-exist, you may see both. This is often reported as being a source of frustration among patients who suspect their problems to be triggered by certain foods or other allergens, and would therefore prefer to see an allergist with an understanding of intolerance, so that either or both possibilities can be considered.

Eczema and asthma can be caused by other factors which lung and skin specialists can identify, advise on and prescribe treatment for, but often what the sufferer wants is a dietary or allergen-avoidance solution. Organ-based specialists are unlikely to be the best healthcare professionals to manage a systemic problem mediated by intolerance or allergy.

Allergists

Doctors are not always aware of the nearest available specialist, and this is when the allergy charities can be of invaluable help. Allergy UK, for instance, maintains a database of specialists and clinics working in intolerance and allergy, and can give either patients or GPs their contacts. The same applies if there is no specialist in the area covered by your primary care trust (PCT), or if a referral is for some reason denied.

Gastroenterologists

When complaints are confined to the digestive system, you may be referred to a gastroenterologist to rule out more serious conditions. There are many tests you may undergo.

Barium x-ray tests

These allow the examination of your gastro-intestinal tract for structural abnormalities or blockages. They employ a barium compound which shows up clearly under X-ray.

A barium swallow involves drinking a solution of barium sulphate while pictures are taken of your upper body; it's intended to detect swallowing disorders, oesophagal abnormalities and causes of chronic heartburn.

A barium meal takes longer. After drinking the solution, you lie down while X-rays are taken of your stomach and small intestine.

A barium enema is administered rectally. The solution coats the rectum and colon, allowing them to be viewed under X-ray.

Endoscopy

This is an internal examination using a lighted tube (endoscope) passed through your mouth or anus and into various parts of the gastro-intestinal tract. The probe is equipped with a camera, allowing the examiner to check for ulceration, damage or inflammation.

Some endoscopes are equipped with tiny pliers, enabling a small tissue sample, or biopsy, to be taken. For instance, in the event of a positive transglutaminase test, an upper gastro-intestinal endoscopy and biopsy on the gut wall can confirm coeliac disease if the villi are seen to be worn down or flattened.

Bowel transit test

A more scientific, and accurate, way of considering intestinal transit is through a test which monitors the progress of mildly radioactive markers ingested in capsule form. An X-ray taken several days later can reveal how many markers have been excreted and the distribution of those remaining.

Irritable bowel syndrome (IBS)

If a gastroenterologist can find nothing wrong, you may be told it's IBS.

There is no test for IBS. The diagnosis is reached through a combined process of elimination, a comparative analysis of your symptoms set against certain 'qualifying' criteria, and the clinical acumen of your medical officer. Sadly, the condition is ill-understood. It is sometimes missed; occasionally diagnosed in error.

IBS is not a *structural* gut disorder, but a *functional* one, affecting around a third of the population. A 'hypersensitive digestive system', is how some have described it. Many of its manifestations – diarrhoea and/or constipation, abdominal pain, bloating, flatulence, borborygmi – overlap with those of food intolerance, and the two often go hand in hand.

Other symptoms include: urgency to use the loo, passing mucus, changes in frequency and appearance of stools, rectal pain or having to strain during a bowel movement, and erratic, 'false' or incomplete movements.

Possible causes include most of those associated with food intolerance, such as enzyme deficiencies and gut dysbiosis. Alcohol, smoking, medicines or a poor diet can all pose problems. Stress and psychological mechanisms may be major factors. Most sufferers identify their personal bugbears through experience, and self-manage their condition with minimal input from healthcare professionals.

IBS is a real problem which is often related to diet or food intolerance. In perhaps half of cases, it can be helped considerably by dietary modification, but certainly not in all. Accordingly, a consultation with a dietitian may help.

5
Dietitians, elimination diets and IgG

A referral to a dietitian, be it via a doctor or other specialist, is more likely than one to an allergist. However this is not automatic, and there may be a long waiting list. Again, the allergy charities can help find a local dietitian with an interest in intolerance.

What does a dietitian do?

Dietitians translate the science of nutrition into practical, jargon-free advice about food which their patients can use to achieve or maintain optimal health. They are involved in diagnostic processes and the dietary management and treatment of diverse forms of illness. Working one-to-one, they are therefore ideally placed to help the food sensitive.

The private option
For any number of reasons, you may elect to see a dietitian privately. These include: having private healthcare; word-of-mouth recommendation; dissatisfaction with your doctor's opinion; wanting advice on related matters, such as weight management; preference for diet-based over prescription-based treatments.

Ensure your dietitian is state registered – the Health Professions Council hold a database on their website (www.hpc-uk.org/register/index.html). State registered dietitians (SRDs) are qualified specialists subject to rigorously upheld working guidelines and carefully regulated by law.

Beware the alternative therapist also going by the title 'nutritionist' – a term sadly not yet legally protected like 'dietitian'. The British Nutrition Foundation and the Nutrition Society are among those pressing for such a safeguard to be conferred, but until then, expect its occasional misappropriation by unqualified individuals to persist.

Consultations
An initial consultation can last up to an hour. You will be asked about your home life, working life, diet, relationship with food, symptoms and medical history.

If you have come with a detailed referral letter and clear

diagnosis, such as of coeliac disease, your dietitian will work with you to formulate a suitable eating and lifestyle plan. If you have come with an undefined problem, the initial consultation will be geared towards diagnosis. Before considering intolerance, your dietitian may seek to rule out other possibilities, such as food aversion (Chapter 12).

Sometimes, a healthy-eating plan may be advised. If your diet is rich in processed foods, you could be suffering from the unglamorous condition of undernutrition – so you may be asked to avoid ready meals, takeaways, refined carbohydrates and so on, while increasing your intake of fruits, vegetables, fish and complex carbohydrates.

But if your diet is generally healthy, your dietitian may suggest an elimination diet.

Elimination diets

Sometimes called exclusion diets, these diagnostic diets are founded on a simple rationale: to remove from your diet all the foods under suspicion and give your body respite from them until symptoms clear up; then, once you've improved, to reintroduce – and thereby 'challenge' – the foods individually, while symptoms are closely monitored to identify possible triggers.

Accordingly, in all but the simplest elimination diets, there is an *exclusion* period – lasting two to six weeks – and a *reintroduction* period of perhaps several months. In the absence of a guaranteed test for food intolerance, this approach is currently the best available. Doctors and allergists, as well as dietitians, may use it.

There are four basic types, outlined below in ascending order of stringency, the more rigorous ones sometimes being used once a milder version has failed. Usually, the less restrictive the diet, the longer the initial period of exclusion.

Simple elimination diet

Here, only one food or group is excluded, typically the dairy suite of foods. If symptoms clear after a month or so, a food 'challenge' can be used to confirm the dairy intolerance.

Multiple elimination diet

The most common diet. There are variations, but many practitioners adopt customized versions of the Addenbrooke's Diet template, devised by Dr John Hunter at the well-known hospital in Cambridge, England, after which it is named.

Multiple elimination diets usually exclude many or all of the foods most commonly implicated in food sensitivities, namely wheat and grains, all dairy produce, eggs, yeast, sugar, alcohol and caffeine. Often, spicy or smoked or mature foods may be deemed off limits, as well as some fruits (often citrus fruits), soya or meats.

Few foods diet

Usually attempted only on desperate patients enduring chronic, severe and systemic problems, with dozens of suspects. One fat and protein source (for example, lamb or turkey), one carbohydrate food (rice or potatoes), one source of vitamins (pears) and still mineral water are permitted during exclusion – and nothing else. The diet demands enormous willpower and motivation.

Elemental diet

Used exceptionally, this is based on pre-digested food formulas which in theory are free of possible offenders. Patients on elemental diets need considerable professional supervision and support, not least because the taste of the formulas is notoriously diabolical.

Preparation

On prescribing a diagnostic elimination diet, your dietitian will explain what will be required of you – the importance of sticking to the plan, how to avoid 'hidden' forms of the excluded foods, and which 'replacement' foods to eat (such as rice milk for dairy milk). Although devoted largely to those *diagnosed* with the relevant food intolerances, Chapters 6 to 9 offer further advice about food substitutes, while Chapter 13 has practical tips about living on a restricted diet.

Your diet should not be undertaken without preparation: choose a largely empty period in your social calendar; plan to start on a Saturday, when work worries are far from your mind; get into the 'food diary' mindset a week before you begin; stock up on permitted foods; give away any eliminated foods in stock which may tempt you to stray; recruit the support of family and friends; plan what you will be eating and doing on the first few days of the diet; get into the habit of checking food labels.

The exclusion period

Sometimes called the withdrawal or elimination phase, this first stage can be dull, unpleasant and stressful. One problem is craving an absent food. This is normal, and considered by many a sign that the food is problematic.

Do be patient. It is unlikely you'll experience immediate relief, and you may feel worse initially. Stay motivated by reminding yourself that: this diet is temporary, and soon you'll be able to reintroduce some favourite foods; it is likely that you *will* find out what has been causing you problems; when that happens, you'll be able to take steps to return to good health.

If there is no improvement during this period, then you and your dietitian must consider the possibility that the unknown culprits were not excluded, that you have a psychological reaction to food, or that food sensitivity is not the problem. The last case can be deeply frustrating, but you should consider this at least a partial success, in that you have eliminated food as the cause of your ill-health. Return immediately to your doctor. Do not give up looking for a solution.

The reintroduction period

This is when you sequentially 'challenge' your body with individual foods, and is usually begun a few days after your symptoms have improved substantially or disappeared. Your dietitian will advise.

Work through the list of foods you have been given, reintroducing one every three or four days, or as regularly as prescribed, keeping your food diary updated constantly. Introduce a normal portion of the food, and provided there is no reaction, eat it on the following day too.

If after three or four days your symptoms have not returned, you can reincorporate the food into your diet – taking care not to come to rely on it heavily – and introduce the next food on your list in a similar manner. And so on.

Following the withdrawal phase, your body can become more attuned to foods that disagree with it, so much so that when you happen to reintroduce one, the response time may be reduced and the intensity of the symptom greater – a powerful indicator of intolerance.

Your dietitian will prepare you for this, and tell you what to do. Obviously, stop eating the food, and wait until all symptoms disappear again. If your reaction was not severe, some dietitians may suggest you retest the food to confirm the intolerance. If not, continue to work down the list.

Results

If you reach the end of the diet having reintroduced everything you were eating previously without any adverse effects, then you can consider yourself – at least for now – cured. Perhaps all your body needed was a 'break' from certain foods, and the diet provided it. Unfortunately, though, you won't have learned what those foods were, so there is always a possibility of reinvoking the intolerance in future. See Chapter 14 for advice.

Any foods you have reacted to will need to be removed from your diet. Your dietitian will advise on your subsequent 'maintenance' restricted diet and will want to re-evaluate your health periodically over the coming months.

Don't be disheartened if your favourite foods are among those removed. Many intolerances are not permanent (coeliac disease being a glaring exception), and after between three and twelve months' abstinence, the foods can usually be gradually reintroduced.

Key points about elimination diets

They are *diagnostic*, used by health professionals for short periods with the exclusive intention of identifying problem foods; they're *not* quick-fix 'detoxes' or weight-loss plans.

They should only be attempted under a dietitian's guidance and with a doctor's approval.

If you think you can't adhere to your plan, tell your dietitian straight away – she may be able to give you leeway without compromising the integrity of the diagnostic process.

It goes without saying that all foods to which you are classically allergic should be avoided.

If something goes wrong – you get sick or accidentally eat an off-limits food – tell your dietitian at once, as she will advise on the best action. It is unlikely that all will be lost.

Alternative tests

As diagnostic aids, elimination diets are drawn out and laborious and therefore cannot suit everybody. Which makes the availability of declared 'tests' for food intolerance appealing to those who, not unreasonably, want a quick solution.

These tests are not available on the NHS. Some are expensive. Many are bizarre and quite empty of scientific virtue or merit. All are clinically unvalidated.

We will briefly consider only the most common below.

Electrodermal/Vega testing

Perhaps the most well-known, sold widely by fringe practitioners. The Vega employs an electrical circuit to measure minute changes in skin resistance when exposed to test substances. Quantum, BEST,

Dermatron and LISTEN are alternative, modernized or computerized versions of electrodermal testing.

Pulse testing

Readings are taken before and after exposure to test substances. An increased 'after' rate is purportedly indicative of sensitivity.

Kinesiology

Highly subjective procedure whereby test substances are placed in the patient's mouth or hands; the practitioner then manipulates the subject's limbs to ascertain whether muscular strength reduces.

Hair analysis

Hair samples are examined for low mineral levels, from which conclusions are drawn about the body's deficiencies and, consequently, sensitivities.

Leucocytotoxic testing

Here, food extracts are mixed with a patient's blood cells and later examined under a microscope – cellular distortion is deemed diagnostic of sensitivity. The ALCAT and NuTron tests are versions of leucocytotoxic testing.

Iridology

A diagnosis is formulated on the basis of examining specific areas of the eye's iris.

Other tests that someone, somewhere, saw fit to invent include those which employ fingernail analyses, dowsing rods, swinging pendulums and – in case you thought matters couldn't get any more absurd (or potentially dangerous) – injections of urine.

Many bodies, including the British Nutrition Foundation and the British Dietetic Association, have voiced deep concern about the availability of such tests. Studies published in the *British Medical Journal* have failed to find any diagnostic value in many, including Vega. The British Society for Allergy and Clinical Immunology and the Royal College of Physicians have dismissed a host as wholly unreliable. SRDs and allergists will never work with them or formulate elimination diets on results derived from them. The allergy charities warn against them.

Remember – misdiagnosis by a non-qualified practitioner using a non-validated test can not only lead to inappropriate dietary exclusions, but also increase the likelihood of a genuine medical condition being overlooked.

IgG-antibody testing

In a sense there is little controversy about the tests considered above, because they are almost unanimously rejected within medical and dietetic circles. What *has* polarized today's scientific brains, is IgG testing.

IgG antibodies to foods form when undigested proteins pass through the gut wall and into the bloodstream, where they are set upon by the immune system. In large numbers, these IgG antibodies may have an inflammatory or possibly 'toxic' effect and can activate other parts of the immune system to induce a catalogue of symptoms.

In recent years, private IgG testing has been revolutionized by **YORK**TEST Laboratories (see Useful addresses), whose *food*SCAN tests exploit a method known as the enzyme-linked immunosorbent assay (ELISA) to analyse a sample of blood for IgGs to food proteins.

It is not the accuracy of the test itself that is in dispute, but the presupposition that IgG antibodies are guilty of provoking symptoms.

Detractors rightly point out IgG antibodies to food are found in all individuals to varying degrees, the greater proportion of whom are not reporting symptoms of food intolerance. Therefore the presence of IgGs cannot be deemed diagnostic of intolerance, but rather markers of exposure to foods typical of the individual's diet.

The counterargument is this. Those who report symptoms of food intolerance may be more susceptible to excess IgG antibodies or have immune systems which are more sensitive to them. By identifying these IgGs, the culprit foods can be excluded and the reactions reduced or eliminated. Research is ongoing in this area, but support for the IgG theory is strengthening.

The tests

YORKTEST's IgG testing essentially offers an alternative to the diagnostic elimination diet. If you opt for it, you will be sent a food intolerance indicator kit, which you can use to take a pinprick of your blood to send to the laboratory for examination. The kits are also available from some chemists.

A simple and inexpensive yes/no test will let you know whether or not you have raised IgG antibodies. In the event of a 'yes', subsequent quantitative tests can assess specific IgGs to over forty common foods (around £135) or over 110 foods (around £230).

Results are presented in three categories:

- No Reaction – foods you can eat freely;
- Rotate – foods to which you have a moderate reaction, and that you should eat only once every four days;
- Avoid – foods which you should exclude for an extended period dependent on the scale of matching IgG in the blood.

You will also receive a telephone consultation with a nutritionist to develop a suitable maintenance diet plan based on the results, literature containing comprehensive support information, and a year's membership to Allergy UK.

Again, the following four chapters will help you with specific food exclusions, while Chapter 13 advises more generally about living on a restricted diet and later reintroducing foods.

Success rates

There are acknowledged limitations to the test. Reactions not due to IgG-mediated mechanisms – such as coeliac disease, pharmacological responses or food aversions – are not identified. Because antibodies only form to proteins, any reactions to carbohydrates or fats will not be picked up either.

However, independent surveys of patients taking the test and following the dietary recommendations based on the results suggest that over 70% derive significant symptomatic relief from it.

IgG and IBS

The results of an independent double-blind clinical trial conducted at the University Hospital of South Manchester, and published in the journal *Gut* in October 2004, suggest that a similar elimination diet based on elevated IgG antibodies can significantly reduce symptoms of IBS.

IBS sufferers taking the *food*SCAN are offered a year's membership to the IBS Network rather than to Allergy UK.

Precautions

Always check with your doctor before starting any diet plan. This is especially important if you are on any medication, perhaps for asthma or diabetes. In rare cases, some foods can interfere with certain medicines, so if you are making rigorous modifications this could have consequences. Other situations where you should unquestionably obtain medical approval include recent illness, young or old age, or pregnancy.

6

Gluten, wheat and grains

If you were to embark upon a diet rich in chocolate, eating it as a substantial part of all your meals, you would probably soon feel very unwell. If you were then to stop consuming chocolate and revert to a healthy regimen, your nausea would fade. Would such symptomatic relief indicate a chocolate intolerance? Almost certainly not. It would simply mean you have been eating too much chocolate. In all probability, you could continue to eat chocolate – moderately – as part of a healthy diet.

We in the West follow a diet rich in gluten and wheat. This undoubtedly provokes numerous symptoms in some people. Abruptly adopting a no-gluten, no-wheat policy may well relieve those symptoms, but that does not necessarily mean the individuals concerned are intolerant to either or both – it can merely signify that they have been eating too much, and that they benefit from cutting back.

Others may need to curb their consumption for a short period. Often, an elimination diet will reveal a strong reaction to wheat, while a positive IgG antibody test may also indicate the possible benefit of restricting it for up to a year.

And for a few – principally, coeliac sufferers – lifelong exclusion of gluten is imperative.

Gluten

True gluten is the dominant mix of proteins found in wheat – proteins such as glutenin, globulin, albumin and gliadin. It is the gliadin fraction of gluten which is understood to cause the toxic auto-immune response that corrodes the intestinal lining of coeliacs.

Proteins analagous to gliadin are present in rye, barley and oats and go by the names of secalin, hordein and avenin respectively, while some less common grains such as kamut and spelt (both ancient forms of wheat) and triticale (a cross between wheat and rye) contain related proteins.

The definition of gluten has been broadened to encompass all these groups of grain proteins which coeliacs should avoid.

Living with coeliac's

Symptoms of coeliac disease can vary not only in nature but also in severity – so much so that mild tiredness, digestive troubles and skin problems, for instance, may simply be tolerated, misdiagnosed as IBS or wheat intolerance, or missed altogether by doctors unfamiliar with the various presentations of the illness. Consequently, diagnosis is commonly made at an advanced age, often in middle or late adulthood, and can come as a shock.

Around a quarter of a million people in the UK are diagnosed coeliacs, but there may be as many as half a million unaware of their condition, as the estimate of sufferers now stands at 1% of the population. If you're a coeliac, you're certainly not alone.

Excluding gluten is a formidable undertaking. Aside from the obvious sources of bread, pasta, cakes, biscuits and many cereals, 'hidden' gluten can be found in such products as stock cubes, sausages, cheese spreads and soups – largely because of wheat's supplementary roles in food production as thickener or stabilizer.

The lists below, while not exhaustive, give you a fair summary of what you can and cannot eat as a coeliac. Unfortunately, no list can be 100% reliable, as there is always the risk of a normally safe product being produced by a particular manufacturer using non-gluten-free ingredients. Conscientious label reading is paramount.

The most current information is available from the excellent support charity Coeliac UK (see Useful Addresses). Its regularly updated *Gluten-Free Food & Drink Directory* contains over 11,000 food products.

Foods and ingredients containing gluten

Grains, flours and starches

Wheat, wheatgerm, wheat bran, bulgur wheat, durum wheat, semolina, couscous; barley, rye, oats, spelt, kamut, triticale. Most flours and starches made from these grains.

Bakery and pastas

All ordinary breads, breadsticks, doughs, cakes, biscuits, pastries, pastas and noodles made from the above grains and flours.

Cereals

Wheat-based cereals such as shredded wheat, brans, wheat flakes and ground wheat farina; mueslis, flaked or porridge oats, barley and rye flakes.

Meat and fish products

Meat pies, pasties and burgers, sausages, some salamis, tinned meats, pâtés and meat pastes, breaded meats, fishcakes, fish fingers, battered fish, many fish pastes.

Vegetable products

Breaded vegetables, vegetarian pâtés, some tinned vegetables and soups.

Dairy products

Some processed cheeses, cheese spreads and thickened milks and creams.

Drinks

Beers, ales, lagers; whisky, bourbon and other grain spirits; most malted drinks; barley waters; some coffee substitutes and hot instant drinks.

Miscellany

Stock cubes, gravy granules/mixes, white/malt vinegar, soy sauce and other condiments or blended seasonings, confectionery (some chocolate bars, sweets, chewing gum and liquorice, for instance), savoury snacks, some medicines.

'Hidden' ingredients

Some food starches and modified starches; cereal binder, filler or protein; malt extract.

Foods and ingredients free of gluten

Grains, flours and starches

Rice, maize/corn, millet, buckwheat, quinoa, sorghum, teff. Flours and starches made from these and from soya, chickpeas, lentils, tapioca, potatoes and other roots. (NB: Confusingly, potato flour is sometimes called farina, a word also used to describe a form of wheat cereal.)

Bakery and pastas

All specially made gluten-free breads, cakes, biscuits, pastas and noodles made from these grains and flours and/or other gluten-free ingredients.

Cereals

Corn flakes; rice cereals.

Meat and fish products

Fresh meat, some tinned meats; fresh fish and most tinned fish.

Vegetable and fruit products

All fresh and frozen vegetables, pulses, salads and all fruits.

Dairy products

All milks, creams, butters, yoghurts, unprocessed cheeses.

Drinks

Pure fruit and vegetable juices, most wines, brandy, potato vodkas, tequila, rum.

Miscellany

Nuts, seeds, eggs, pure chocolate, herbs, pure spices, vegetable oils, margarines, cider/wine vinegars.

'Hidden' ingredients

Codex wheat starch (wheat starch with virtually all gluten removed); maltodextrin; wheat-derived glucose syrup; hydrolyzed or textured vegetable protein (HVP/TVP).

The bad news about coeliac's ...

- *You must adhere strictly to the gluten-free diet.* Even a tiny amount can be extremely harmful. Non-compliance can lead to further damage to the intestinal lining, in the long term increasing your risk of complications such as lymphomas. Your gut can heal itself only a finite number of times.
- *You must read all labels.* Gluten can be hidden in innocent-looking foods. Beware products 'dusted' with flours (such as chewing gums) and those with added flour (some powdered spices, for instance). Watch for ambiguity, too: 'food starch' could be wheat starch (perhaps not gluten-free) or corn starch (gluten-free) while terms such as 'natural flavouring' are frustratingly vague. When in doubt, avoid.
- *There is conflicting anecdotal information on certain foods.* Some coeliacs tolerate rye-based spirits and malt vinegars, for instance, while others believe them toxic. If in doubt, seek your dietitian's advice or avoid altogether, as experimenting with products can be risky.

- *You need to exercise constant vigilance with 'false friends'.* Pure cider, for instance, is gluten-free, but a malt beverage with apple flavouring going by the name of cider may not be; likewise, tortilla chips should be made from corn, but may be made from wheat.

... and the good

- *Gluten-free foods are now widely available.* You can find them in all supermarkets, healthfood stores and by mail order from specialist companies.
- *Labels are being made increasingly coeliac-friendly.* Many now clearly indicate either 'gluten free' or 'contains gluten'. Several 'no gluten' symbols, depicting a panicle of wheat with a line across it, are also used.
- *Other intolerances* – such as lactose intolerance – which you may have endured as an undiagnosed coeliac should clear up within a year, as the damage the villi in your gut have suffered by a lifetime of gluten consumption is reversed.
- *Some coeliacs may be able to consume modest portions of pure oats.* Discuss this with your healthcare provider first.
- *A selection of some* 200 gluten-free foods is available on prescription.
- *All diagnosed coeliacs are entitled to membership of Coeliac UK*, an invaluable source of information and support.

Other gluten sensitivities

Dermatitis herpetiformis (DH) is a skin condition caused by gluten consumption that is characterized by intensely itchy, blistery and reddened skin patches, usually on the elbows, knees, buttocks and scalp. Many DH sufferers have coeliac disease and a few coeliacs have DH, but either can and does present independently of the other. Medication is available for DH, but a gluten-free diet often removes the need for it, although it may take a year or more for the rashes to clear.

Non-coeliac gluten intolerance is a debated issue. Anecdotal evidence suggests some non-coeliac sufferers of undiagnosed food intolerances improve on a gluten-free diet, but this may be because such a restriction forces dietary experimentation upon an individual, which in itself could confer health benefits – whether subjectively felt or genuine.

There have been a few instances of patients experiencing inflammatory gut reactions to gluten without the villial flattening characteristic of coeliac disease, while gluten-sensitive diarrhoea and mouth ulcers have also been recorded.

Gluten is a complex of proteins and certainly not the easiest substance to digest, so it isn't unfeasible that enzyme deficiencies could be responsible for some adverse responses, especially when there is a localized inflammatory reaction in the gut which increases permeability. A positive IgG test to gluten (or gliadin) might be suggestive of such an intolerance. Other nutritionists have postulated that high gluten intake can slow intestinal transit, thereby posing other problems such as constipation and gut dysbiosis.

More research is needed. If gluten *is* an occasional problem for non coeliacs, then it is unlikely that long-term elimination is required, or indeed to be recommended given that it is, after all, a nutritious protein. Exclusion and then gentle reintroduction after a period of up to a year should permanently resolve most cases.

Many individuals who believe themselves gluten-sensitive may in fact be suffering from: a reaction to yeast, especially if pasta is well tolerated and bread is not (see Chapter 8); a food aversion (Chapter 12); or a response to a non-gluten element of the grain, probably the starch. In this third scenario, the guilty grain is usually wheat.

Wheat

It has been a feature of the human diet for almost 10,000 years and is the dominant grain in the West. It is the main ingredient in a range of foods, such as bread, cereals and pasta, and has a subsidiary role as a binder or 'filler' in many meat, fish and vegetable products. It is versatile, popular and tasty – so why is wheat such a problem food for many?

A lot of wheat is too much wheat, according to the anti-wheat brigade, usually only too ready to point out that the cereal is no longer the pure food it once was. Wheat farming is criticized for its use of pesticides, while the harvested grain itself is often treated to a blitz of mechanical and chemical processing – which sees it stripped of its beneficial wheatgerm and wheat bran, put through a refining process and subjected to a cocktail of preservatives and bleaches. By the time it reaches our shelves as white bread, many of wheat's original vitamins and minerals have been lost.

Not surprisingly, the wheat industry's response to this sort of attack is strong – emphasizing that statutory fortification of white flour boosts its iron, calcium and B vitamin content. 'Wheat is good' remains the core message – along with the not unreasonable reminder that media coverage of wheat sensitivities is often alarmist and inaccurate.

However, the (industry-funded) Grain Information Service says that, coeliacs excluded, only around 0.1% of the population is wheat sensitive, a figure which appears irrationally low in light of all the available evidence and which makes somewhat of a mockery of one of the GIS's website addresses – www.wheatintolerance.co.uk.

Impartial advice on wheat is hard to come by. But the plain truths are these:

- most people do not react adversely to moderate portions of wheat or wheat products;
- many who eat wheat several times a day would probably benefit from replacing a portion of their intake with equally nutritious grains and other sensible food choices;
- the genuinely wheat intolerant should be helped immensely by a variable period of wheat exclusion, followed by a gradual reintroduction to eating nutritious wheat products;
- unless you have coeliac disease or an exceptionally rare wheat allergy, the likelihood of your having to remove wheat permanently from your diet is tiny.

Reactions to wheat

Non-coeliac, non-gluten wheat intolerances are quite common. They respond to reduced dietary intake or a period of exclusion.

Other wheat proteins

It is possible that non-glutenous proteins in wheat may be responsible for some symptoms; a positive IgG to wheat is a common result. Other reports of adverse responses to untoasted but not toasted bread might be explained by a particular protein's reactive capacity being neutralized by a sudden burst of intense heat – but this is conjecture. Different proteins in varying proportions are found in the wheat kernel, wheat bran and wheatgerm, so you may be able to tolerate white flour and bread (made from the wheat kernel) but not bran or wholewheat products – or indeed vice versa.

Wheat fibre and IBS

Complex carbohydrates in wholewheat bread and bran cereals remain the most likely triggers to many reported wheat intolerances. This is especially true for IBS sufferers, when the general advice with regard to wheat and other fibres, dependent on dominant symptoms is:

- with diarrhoea, lower your fibre intake;
- with constipation in the absence of bloating, up your fibre (and fluid) intake;
- with constipation and bloating, lower your fibre intake.

Following these basic guidelines, possibly by adjusting your wholewheat intake, generally produces good results in around 50% of IBS sufferers, so much so that there may be no need for further dietary modifications.

Overeating, bloating and fermentation

Eating too much wheat can lead to bloating – a large plate of al dente pasta, for instance, will continue to absorb water and swell in the gut. Have a smaller portion, as many Italians do.

Too much wholewheat food can present problems too, because it is high in insoluble fibre, an occasional colonic irritant. In some individuals – both with IBS and without – imbalances of gut flora may be causing overfermentation of excess wheat fibre in the bowel, leading to severe bloating and wind – the two main symptoms. Lowering fibre intake for several weeks, thereby allowing flora levels to reset themselves, usually rectifies this problem, providing reintroduction is gentle at first, and large portions of wheat are permanently avoided.

There is another possibility. In the event of brush border enzyme deficiencies in the small intestine, complex carbohydrates may be inadequately broken down, and the incompletely digested sugars which result will not be absorbed by the body. Instead, these may travel on to the colon, where even a balanced gut flora population may ferment them, producing abdominal symptoms such as diarrhoea, bloating and flatulence. (See Chapter 8 for more on the possible effects of simple carbohydrates in the lower digestive tract.) Fermentation in the bowel is a natural and healthy process, and whether all reactions caused by 'overfermentation' should be termed intolerances is moot.

Wheat elimination

Your dietitian or nutritionist will advise you carefully about eliminating wheat, but the following may help:

You should avoid most of the glutenous foods listed on page 51, except rye, barley, oats, and products derived from them or containing them, unless you're also intolerant to these grains. If you are not, wheat elimination is easier. You can eat pure rye bread, for instance, while rye flakes can be taken in muesli or cereals. But take care not to come to depend heavily on rye, as you could risk forming an intolerance to it. Always read labels on rye-based foods to ensure there is no added wheat.

You can eat all the gluten-free foods on page 52, except foods containing or made from Codex wheat starch. The more unusual gluten-free grains – millet, amaranth, quinoa – make nutritious alternative options, and experimenting with them is important; you shouldn't rely on only rice and potatoes, for instance.

Wheat provides protein, fibre, iron, calcium and B vitamins. A mix of alternative grains and foods ought to compensate, but these nutrients are also available from other sources:

- Meats, fish, cheeses, pulses and nuts are rich in *protein.*
- Fruit and vegetables, especially pulses and beans, are rich in *fibre.*
- Meats, fish, pulses, seeds, chocolate and dark dried fruits are rich in *iron.*
- Dairy products, soya milk, bony fish, nuts, seeds and green vegetables are rich in *calcium.*
- Fruit, vegetables, dairy products, fish, meats, nuts, eggs and yeast extracts are rich in *B vitamins.*

Other grain sensitivities

Reactions to other grains are less common. Intolerance to rye is the most likely. If you're sensitive to this grain, avoid all rye breads, such as pumpernickel, and rye crackers. Also check mueslis and cereals for rye content.

If you react to barley, eliminate foods such as any malted products and many beers.

Porridges, mueslis and cereal bars are your principal foes if you are oat sensitive.

Intolerance to rice, not a gluten grain of course, is only common in countries where it is grown and forms a dietary staple. Rice and rice flour products (in rice noodles, for instance) are easily avoided.

7

Milk, dairy and eggs

Cows' milk is a food nature designed to help nurture baby calves. Egg is a food nature designed to help nurture embryonic chicks. Neither food is designed to help nurture human beings. Which might at least in part explain why adverse sensitivities to dairy produce and eggs are so remarkably common in the western world – human digestive systems aren't the foods' intended recipients.

Lactose intolerance

Sometimes called alactasia or hypolactasia, lactose intolerance is the inability to digest lactose – the natural carbohydrate found in all mammalian milks and milk products – and is the most common food intolerance in the world. The condition is caused by a deficiency in the enzyme lactase, required to break lactose down into the simple sugars glucose and galactose.

Undigested lactose cannot be absorbed or metabolized. Instead, it attracts water by osmosis and passes rapidly through the intestinal system, eventually reaching the main colonies of colonic bacteria, which readily feast on the sugar and ferment it, forming fatty acids and waste gases. These processes are responsible for the symptoms associated with lactose intolerance, which can manifest themselves as rapidly as half an hour after consumption. The symptoms are borborygmi, bloating and abdominal pain, excessive flatulence and frothy diarrhoea.

There are two different forms of lactose intolerance. *Primary lactose intolerance (primary lactase deficiency)* is the inherited form, which usually presents between the ages of five and twenty, when lactase production begins to decrease naturally. This reduction can be partial, in which case the consumption of a certain 'safe' quantity of dairy produce will be tolerated, or it can be almost total, when symptoms may be triggered by nothing more than a splash of milk in a mug of coffee. Primary lactose intolerance is permanent.

Secondary lactose intolerance (secondary lactase deficiency) is a transient condition caused by damage to the lactase-producing brush border sites in the small intestine. It can effect anybody, at any age. Typically, the gut lining will have been injured by a bout of gastroenteritis, but Crohn's disease, untreated coeliac disease, recent bowel surgery, alcohol abuse or undernutrition can be to blame. The condition usually goes into remission following a month or so of a dairy-free diet, once the jejunal wall has recovered.

Prevalence

Around 70 to 75% of the world's population is lactose intolerant, with rates varying dramatically among different ethnic groups. The lowest rates are seen in northern and western Europe. Dairy farming is ideally suited to the temperate climates typical of this region, where it has been an established practice for centuries. Accordingly, these Europeans have largely 'held on' to their ability to digest lactose. Only around 5% are lactase deficient.

Elsewhere in the world, the picture is very different. Eastern and Mediterranean Europeans and Latin Americans, for instance, show higher rates. In tropical climates, where dairy farming is generally absent and where milks and cheeses do not form part of the regular diet, the ability to digest lactose throughout life has largely disappeared. This is particularly true of many Asian or black African populations, among which rates of adult lactose intolerance can approach 100%. Some exceptions are Mongols and African Fulani, Tuareg and Tutsi peoples.

Treatment

The symptoms of lactose intolerance may be temporarily unpleasant, but the condition is harmless. Only when symptomatic diarrhoea is heavy might nutrient absorption be compromised – accordingly, extreme lactose intolerants should not persist with consuming quantities of dairy products and putting up with the consequences regardless.

Any 'treatment' is largely dependent on the level of inconvenience and discomfort you endure from your current dairy consumption. In mild cases, an only slightly reduced dietary intake of dairy products may be required, something unlikely to adversely affect your nutrition. More sensitive individuals may like to take greater evasive measures, or even exclude dairy foods altogether. Your dietitian can advise.

For most lactose intolerants, it's possible through trial and error to establish a daily limit at or below which no adverse symptoms are felt – although you may have to review this as you get older, as lactase production decreases with age.

Foods which contain lactose include:

- all varieties of cows', sheep's and goats' milks, reduced-fat milks, heat-treated milks and powdered milks;
- hard cheeses, soft cheeses and cottage cheeses;
- creams, yoghurts, ice creams, butters, custards, etc.;
- sweet baked products, such as cakes and croissants;
- white and milk chocolates.

Foods which *may* contain lactose include:

- breads and savoury baked products (especially in the USA);
- ready-made meals, such as curries;
- soups (typically 'cream of' soups);
- sauces (some Italian or Indian sauces, for instance);
- dips, spreads and dressings;
- convenience products, such as instant mashes;
- confectionery, desserts;
- instant hot drinks and sweeteners;
- medicines and tablets.

Note that the additive antioxidants and acidity regulators E325–E329 – the lactates – and the sugar lactitol (E966) are generally milk-derived and may affect you.

Other terms to look out for on labelling include milk solids, or curds/casein, and milk liquids, or whey, which signify unpredictable quantities of lactose in the product. Specific milk whey proteins which are sometimes listed separately on ingredients, such as lactalbumin, lactoglobulin and ovalbumin, should in theory be free of lactose, but this may not be the case in practice.

All this may seem quite daunting, particularly if you delight in dairy foods. But lactase deficiency need not impose insufferable limitations on you, as the lactose content in various foods varies widely. For instance, most mature or hard cheeses – such as Cheddar, Stilton, Edam and Parmesan – are naturally low in lactose and may be well-tolerated; ditto full-fat soft cheeses, such as Philadelphia.

Live yoghurt is another food which could agree with you, because it contains lactobacilli bacteria (such as *lactobacillus acidophillus* and *lactobacillus bulgaricus*) which take over the job of lactose digestion for you. Dietary intake of these so-called 'friendly' bacteria is said to replenesh colonies already living in your intestinal tract, and help in digesting lactose when the body's lactase production is insufficient.

Fattier products and those of a thicker consistency are generally better tolerated because they tend to slow down gastric emptying and subsequent intestinal transit, increasing the likelihood of more thorough lactose digestion. This is why full-fat cheeses appear to be more tolerable to the lactase deficient; and there is also some evidence to suggest full-fat milks are better handled than skimmed varieties. Butter, too, is rarely a problem, as it is principally fat. Logically, dairy products consumed as part of a meal, not separately or on an empty stomach, are more likely to be adequately digested.

Reduced or low-lactose milks, such as Lactolite, are worth trying. Lactose levels in these do vary, though, so always read the label.

Those who wish to continue to eat the range of dairy products should talk to their doctor about the possibility of taking a digestive enzyme supplement containing lactase to aid with digestion. Liquid lactase preparations to add to milk are also available. Enquire at healthfood stores. (Enzyme supplements should generally be avoided if you have any gastric inflammation or ulceration.)

Additionally, these are entirely free of lactose: all soya milks, yoghurts or 'cheeses'; all milks made from rice, oats, quinoa, almonds, hazelnuts, coconut and potato; all foods labelled 'dairy free' or 'suitable for vegans'; carob bars, and pure, dark chocolate.

Cows' milk protein intolerance (CMPI)

Adverse delayed reactions to milk proteins differ considerably from those to milk sugars, insomuch as dermal symptoms such as urticaria and eczema, and asthma, tiredness and arthritic pain are among the typical responses, rather than the rapid-onset digestive symptoms suggestive of lactose intolerance.

You can be intolerant to either the solid curds (casein) or the liquid whey constituents; in total, there are around twenty proteins in milk with immuno-triggering capacity. In practice, isolating the particular culprit or culprits is impossible via an elimination diet; foodSCAN only delivers results on wholemilk IgG antibodies.

UHT (ultra-heat treated) milk might be better tolerated because the temperature to which it has been subjected (132°C) may denature some of the proteins' antigenic potential. This could also be true of evaporated milk, and possibly even condensed milk; while boiling your own milk may increase your tolerance towards it.

You are unlikely to derive benefit from switching between whole milks or skimmed varieties, but you may be able to handle goats' milk or – more probably – sheep's milk.

Like all reactions to proteins, a period of restriction followed by slow reintroduction is often advised for CMPI. Because they are the richest dairy sources of protein, cheeses are the most likely villains, and will usually be reintroduced last.

Replacement foods

The primary concern in eliminating dairy produce is finding an alternative source of calcium – but this needn't be a problem. Foods rich in this vital mineral include: bony fish; dark green vegetables (broccoli, cabbage, spinach); pulses; whole grains; nuts, seeds and dried fruits; fortified non-dairy milks, yoghurts and cheeses.

If you rely on cheeses for protein, ensure your diet is rich in an appropriate combination of protein-rich meats, fish, wholegrains, pulses, soya products, nuts and seeds.

Dairy – friend or foe?

The situation with dairy mirrors that to wheat. Yes, dairy products are one of the most commonly implicated offenders in food intolerance. But, again, the problem is largely one of overconsumption.

Like wheat, dairy boasts analogous for and against camps. In the 'pro' corner come bodies such as the farmers unions and the Dairy Council, the latter of whom promote a three-portions-a-day policy (one portion being a small chunk of cheese or pot of yoghurt). In the 'no' corner stand the detox diet gurus, and organizations such as PETA (People for the Ethical Treatment of Animals), who campaign for fairer treatment of dairy cows.

Here are the facts:

- milk, yoghurt and cheese are undoubtedly nutritious and convenient sources of calcium, proteins and B vitamins – but these nutrients are by no means exclusive to dairy produce;
- lactose intolerants can often reduce their dairy intake and enjoy a drastic alleviation of symptoms without total exclusion;
- those with CMPI often recover fully following a period of abstinence;
- unless you have severe primary lactose intolerance or a genuine milk allergy, it is unlikely you will need to follow a permanently dairy-free diet (whether you wish to exclude dairy on ethical grounds, or for other health reasons, is of course entirely your call).

Eggs

You can be intolerant to egg yolk proteins, to egg white proteins, or to both. If you are intolerant to chicken egg proteins, a cross reaction with proteins of other birds' eggs is probable.

As with milk, some egg proteins you may be responding adversely to are denatured by heat, so you might react only to raw egg products, rather than cooked. The more comprehensive *food*SCAN tests for IgGs to yolk and white proteins separately.

Egg white intolerance is more common. The reactive proteins in egg white revel in some impressive names, including ovalbumin, ovotransfferin, ovomucin, ovoglobulin and ovovitellin, which are sometimes listed on labels.

The allergenic proteins in egg yolk are apovitellenin I, apovitellenin VI and phosvitin. The additive lecithin (E322), although usually soya-derived, is sometimes produced from yolk.

However, cross-contamination cannot be guaranteed against, so in practice it may be wise to exclude all egg-containing products if you need to eliminate one but not both of egg white or yolk.

Aside from obvious sources – quiches, omelettes, mayonnaises and egg noodles – many prepared foods may also contain egg, so you have to be vigilant. Among these are pastas and pasta sauces (e.g. carbonara); baked goods, such as breads, biscuits, buns, pastries and cakes; desserts, such as custard, puddings, mousses, crème caramel; foods which are breaded or battered; dressings and sauces (e.g. Hollandaise, tartare); confectionery; and 'foam' in drinks such as beers and coffees.

Because eggs are rarely overconsumed, few rely on them as their primary protein source, meaning undernutrition due to egg elimination is unlikely. In recipes, however, eggs may be missed. Egg replacement preparations are available from free-from food suppliers or healthfood stores, but there are plenty of DIY solutions. For instance, when egg is used a glazing agent, substitute either a sugar solution or gelatine, the latter of which also serves as a good setting agent when needed. Try six tablespoons of a fruit juice (citrus or apple) instead of an egg used as a liquefier, and for an excellent binder try apple sauce, soya desserts, tofu or bananas. The wonderful Vegan Society (see Useful addresses) has an abundance of further egg-replacement ideas.

8

Sugars and yeasts

Our tastebuds love sugar, but our bodies are not so keen. Along with its twin evil – saturated fat – refined sugar in the diet is one of the greatest nutritional scourges in the West. Too much has catastrophic consequences – dental erosion and obesity are just two of the best-known legacies.

A third is diabetes, a disease virtually unheard of until last century's boom in the production, availability and consumption of sugar. This illness is worthy of consideration, and not only because the road towards it is scattered with intolerance-like reactions.

Hypoglycaemia and the sugar rush

When we eat and rapidly digest a food rich in ordinary table sugar – that is, sucrose – we enjoy a post-digestive surge of glucose in our blood, which provides the sugar 'high' so beloved of the sweet-toothed. In sugar-sensitive children sometimes unjustly labelled 'hyperactive', this rush may provoke the characteristic symptoms of mischievous, high-spirited or disruptive behaviour.

It is important to the body that blood glucose levels are kept stable. This it manages by releasing insulin, a pancreatic hormone, whose purpose it is to encourage the uptake of glucose by the body's cells.

But following a sudden steep rise in blood glucose, the pancreas 'panics' and releases surplus insulin. Over time, indeed years, the body can react to such overload by developing a 'resistance' to the hormone. This has two eventual consequences: the uptake of glucose by the body's cells is compromised, leading to symptoms of tiredness and low energy; and excess dietary glucose remains in the blood, where it spills over into the urine, causing increased thirst and an urge to pass water. This is type-II diabetes.

Pre-diabetes, surplus insulin release in response to a glucose surge is problematic in itself, because it encourages the uptake of glucose into the body's cells too comprehensively, leading to hypoglycaemia, or low blood sugar. Hypoglycaemia boasts an array of unpleasant symptoms, including tiredness, weakness, irritability, headaches and foggy thinking, which appear from about two hours after consumption of a sugar-rich meal. In severe cases, the body secretes the hormone

65

adrenalin to stimulate the release of sugar reserves, which in turn can precipitate palpitations and a disordered mental state. This 'reactive' hypoglycaemia has been implicated in disruptive behaviour in children, and in panic attacks, aggression and violence in adults.

Hunger is another symptom, as is a craving for sugar – the body's means of signalling a request for glucose equilibrium. Satisfying this and eating more sugar completes the circle, and so restarts the cycle – one from which a lot of us find difficult to escape.

Sugar intolerance

Wanting sugar is normal. It is cheap, ubiquitous and tastes good. Conveniently, you can find it not only in all manner of sweets and soft drinks and desserts, but also added to cereals, tinned vegetables, soups and ready meals. The food industry likes sugar too. So much so that it uses it to fulfil several roles – sweetener, preservative, bulking agent. This versatility is celebrated as a virtue, but sufferers of sugar-related ill-health might disagree.

As might those living with food intolerance. Sugar can contribute towards LGS, compromise natural immunity and encourage dysbiotic growth in the gut. Other refined carbohydrates, stress, drugs, drink and – as we shall see later – dietary yeast do their bit too.

Disaccharide sensitivity

This form of sugar intolerance is extremely common, and in more pronounced cases may cause malabsorption problems and mild nutritional deficiencies. First, some definitions:

Polysaccharides, found in grains, vegetables and fruit, are complex carbohydrates that consist of long chains of simple sugar units. Starches are polysaccharides.

Disaccharides are carbohydrates which consist of two simple sugar molecules bound together. Lactose (milk sugar), sucrose (table sugar) and maltose are all disaccharides. They are digested by the enzymes lactase, sucrase and maltase, collectively known as disaccharidases.

Monosaccharides are the simplest carbohydrates, and consist of single sugar units. Glucose, galactose and fructose are all monosaccharides. Of the carbohydrates, only monosaccharides can be absorbed efficiently into the body through the gut wall and metabolized.

As we touched upon in Chapter 2, the digestion of a polysaccharide such as starch begins in the body with salivary amylase, and continues in the duodenum via enzymes secreted by the pancreas. Starch digested in this way is broken down into the disaccharide maltose.

The body, however, cannot absorb maltose, so must digest it further for it to be of use. To that end, it secretes the enzyme maltase in the small intestine, which dismantles each maltose molecule into its two constituent glucose molecules – the simple monosaccharides which the body can absorb and use for energy.

Disaccharides themselves are common in the western diet. For instance, sucrose is a disaccharide which cannot be metabolized until it is broken down by the enzyme sucrase into the monosaccharides glucose and fructose. Disaccharide sensitivity occurs when the body is deficient in a disaccharidase. We have already encountered it. Lactose deficiency, considered in the previous chapter, is a disaccharide intolerance which leads to bloating, flatulence and diarrhoea when undigested lactose is devoured by colonic bacteria. And, as related in Chapter 6, incomplete digestion and fermentation of wheat starches and their breakdown products can lead to similar symptoms.

Although less common than a lactase deficiency, maltase or sucrase deficiencies are not rare. Either may be congenital (a serious condition, invariably picked up soon after birth and treated by strict dietary manipulation), or may be triggered by damage to the enzyme-secreting sites – possibly due to Crohn's disease, alcohol abuse, gastroenteritis or unhealthy flora populations.

If lactose intolerance has been ruled out, and you react to refined white sugars and flours and products containing them with similar symptoms, then you may have an alternative disaccharidase deficiency (a hydrogen breath test can confirm it). Cutting down on sources of refined carbohydrates is the preferred solution. Sucrase supplements are available to help with sucrose digestion, but this approach is not ideal as it will only encourage you to continue eating sugary foods.

Fructose sensitivity

Fructose is a monosaccharide naturally occurring in fruits, many vegetables and honey. As mentioned earlier, it is the simple sugar which with glucose forms the disaccharide sucrose, or table sugar. Clearly then, it is found in a wide range of foods.

Unlike glucose though, fructose is absorbed slowly by the body, and so is not responsible for inducing a blood sugar high. The uptake and metabolism of fructose in fruits is further moderated by the fibre with which it often comes, making fruit a good choice for most of us. But when consumed in large amounts, either in fruit or bound in sucrose, surplus fructose can remain unabsorbed, passing to the lower gut where it prompts the set of abdominal symptoms common to all sugar sensitivities. Some people whose digestive systems are especially inefficient at absorbing fructose are more prone to this, and suffer adverse responses from relatively modest quantities.

There are claims that as many as one in three people are sensitive in this way, but this is probably an overestimate. Some studies have linked mood swings and emotional disturbances with fructose intolerance. The condition is usually easily managed by avoiding fruit juices and refined sugars, particularly on an empty stomach.

Sugar alcohols

Sometimes called polyols and not 'alcoholic' in the usual ·sense, the sugar alcohols occur in varying quantities in a number of fruits and fruit juices, such as apple. They include sorbitol and mannitol, and have been exploited by the food industry as low-calorie bulk sweeteners for use in sugar-free, diabetic and 'low-carb' foods, since they are very poorly absorbed by all of us. If taken in excess, they too can rapidly loosen the stools.

Yeast dysbiosis

Dysbiosis, an imbalance of gut flora, often co-exists with a sugar intolerance because the presence of either can encourage the manifestation of the other. Candida is the best-known culprit yeast, yet many doctors maintain a sceptical view on the broad spectrum of ills some have apportioned to its excessive presence in the digestive tract. But others disagree, and believe a gastro-intestinal candida problem can indeed provoke a selection of adverse symptoms.

Candida commonly lives in the gut without posing a health threat. It is kept in its place by friendly gut bacteria, and may even confer some benefits. What some researchers in this area suspect, however, is that under certain conditions – compromised immunity, poor nutrition, stress, antibiotic usage – candida can 'switch' into a more malevolant form which can reproduce effectively, penetrate the intestinal lining and release toxins.

The symptoms of so-called candidiasis were briefly considered in Chapter 2, and include lapses of memory, problems of co-ordination and breathing difficulties, as well as rectal itchiness and general abdominal malaise. Women may also have cystitis, thrush and PMS – accepted consequences of a vaginal candida infection which can co-exist with an intestinal one.

Refined or undigested sugars provide a feast for candida. A craving for sweet things is a further clue to a possible problem, as is an urge to eat yeast-rich or fermented foods. The onset of new food sensitivities – possibly because the candida has caused LGS, and undigested proteins are now passing more easily into the bloodstream – is a further bad sign.

The anti-yeast diet

An anti-yeast diet – either a no-sugar diet, or a no-sugar/no-yeast diet – is a pure, wholefood regime designed to starve candida of its preferred food (sugar), reduce the possibility of recolonization (by restricting dietary yeast), and thereby return the gastro-intestinal tract to desirable symbiosis. If sugar or yeast are contributing to your symptoms, you will start to feel better quite quickly, usually within weeks.

You will need to avoid the sugars and simple carbohydrates which nourish yeasts and harmful gut bacteria. Their sources are:

- any obviously sugary foods, such as confectionery, soft drinks, cakes, biscuits and desserts;
- any food labelled sugar (white, brown or invert), dextrose, fructose, glucose, maltose, sucrose, syrup (corn, maple, golden), caramel, treacle or molasses;
- the sugar alcohol sweeteners sorbitol, mannitol and glycerol (E420–E422), isomalt (E953) and maltitol, lactitol and xylitol (E965–E967), typically found in dietetic food products;
- fruit juices and sweet dried fruits;
- refined white flours and products made from them.

Some recommend complete exclusion of dairy produce because of their lactose content, but this may not be necessary unless you are lactase deficient. Live yoghurt, for instance, is normally a wise inclusion.

The lack of 'sweetness' the above eliminations force upon your tastebuds may seem punishing, but you are permitted to eat unshelled nuts and modest amounts of fruit (preferably peeled).

Yeast exclusion is tougher. Sources in the diet include:

- most breads, cakes and baked goods;
- all fermented drinks, such as wines, ales, ciders, beers and lagers;
- yeast-based spreads (e.g. Marmite);
- gravies and stock cubes;
- cheeses, especially ripe, mouldy or blue cheeses;

- fermented soy products, such as soy sauce;
- very ripe fruits and dried/preserved fruits;
- mushrooms, mycoproteins, tofu, and hydrolysed or textured vegetable proteins (TVP/HVP);
- vinegar and vinegared foods (dressings, sauces, pickles);
- malted foods;
- black tea;
- anything labelled brewer's yeast, baker's yeast, or leavening agent.

Admittedly, this is highly restrictive. Here are some yeast-free alternatives: unleavened breads such as many Indian breads and Irish soda breads; many (but certainly not all) crispbreads and crackers; pure spirits (gin, rum and vodka); lemon juice and green tea.

Yeast-rich produce does provide B vitamins, but the no-yeast regimen compels you to eat foods such as lean meats, fish, eggs, grains, nuts, seeds and green vegetables, all of which are rich in them too. Raw vegetables are important, especially if your fruit intake is being restricted.

Include in your diet lots of natural anti-fungal foods, such as herbs, spices, garlic, onions and pumpkin seeds. Increasing your pro and prebiotic intake may help too (see below).

If you improve on the plan, your dietitian will doubtlessly impress upon you the importance of not returning to any former high-sugary ways. You don't have to be a saint; occasional treats are fine. But sensible moderation is the key. Guidelines for daily sugar intake stand at roughly 30g per adult, but no more than 50g for a woman and 60g for a man.

Probiotics

Probiotics are in vogue: handy little pots of milky or yoghurty drinks, teeming with so-called friendly bacteria just waiting to be offered the chance of a new life on the lining of a human gut, where they will hopefully settle, start a big, big family, put paid to the neighbourhood bad guys like those dastardly Candidas down at number 74, and repay their host with all manner of protective benefits.

Sound too good to be true? It may be. Dietary probiotics are founded on a sound enough premise, yet the reality doesn't necessarily live up to the hype. Evidence that the bacteria survive the hostile acidic milieu of the stomach and make it to the latter stages of the gastro-intestinal tract is scant. Proof that any which do arrive unscathed succeed in attaching to the gut wall, rather than get flushed away, is perhaps too much to ask for.

There is no harm in trying probiotics. Live plain yoghurt contains probiotic bacteria, and is a healthful, nourishing and calming food. When it comes to the wide range of drinks now on the shelves, do read labels as some contain sugar – hardly an ideal ingredient when you are looking to improve your gut flora.

Probiotics are also available snugly packaged in a capsule, which some argue ensures their safe passage through the inhospitable gastric cauldron before their release into the ambient small intestine.

Prebiotics

Rather than try to enforce new immigration, why not encourage your current tenants to breed instead?

Prebiotics are carbohydrates which health-giving bacteria present in the bowel love to feed on, and which unfriendly bacteria and yeasts positively dislike. The most effective are the indigestible sugars inulin and fructo-oligosaccharides (FOS), either or both of which are found generously in only a few foods: the allium vegetables (onion, leeks, garlic, shallots), asparagus, Jersualem artichokes, chicory and bananas.

Because of this indigestibility, inulin and FOS-rich foods can trigger flatulence – Jerusalem artichokes are especially famed for the southerly gales which sweep in behind them. But in this case, the temporary discomfort is probably worth it for the benefit to your insides. Indeed the Japanese, well ahead of westerners on prebiotics, fortify many of their foods with FOS.

IgG antibodies

Simple sugars are not proteins, don't have antigenic potential, and hence antibodies cannot form to them. This is a common source of misinformation in the press; even food and health magazines have been known to talk erroneously about 'sugar allergies'. For all its other misdemeanours, sugar is not an allergen, and therefore cannot directly antagonize an immune system response.

But IgG antibodies to both brewer's yeast (used in wines and beers) and baker's yeast (in breads) are possible, and detectable by the *food*SCAN. Elimination of all yeast-containing foods for at least three months is the usual recommendation.

9

Meats, fish, vegetables and fruit

Responses to meats, fish and fresh produce are more infrequent than those to foods considered in the previous chapters.

YORKTEST's IgG *food***SCAN** tests against a long gastronomic menu, including duck, haricot bean, cinnamon and carob, and a quirkier intolerance may be identified on an elimination diet too. But such reactions seldom occur. In the event of a positive in either case, such foods can typically be removed from the diet without difficulty or detrimental nutritional consequences.

Other foods, however, may inconvenience you more. They are considered here in rough order of prevalence.

Soya

Responses to the soya bean and its many products and derivatives are increasingly common. Vegans and vegetarians are the most likely to find soya exclusion arduous, because of the bean's widespread use as a milk, protein and meat alternative. Coeliacs, too, may have difficulty, given that soya flour is often used as a wheat flour replacement.

Soya products can crop up anywhere. Here is what you will need to exclude:

- most vegan/vegetarian burgers, pies, sausages and prepared meals;
- soya milks, cheeses and yoghurts;
- fermented soya products, such as soya sauce, tofu, tempeh and miso;
- any food labelled soya flour, soya protein, vegetable proteins (HVP/TVP), vegetable starch or gum (they are usually soya), soya caseinate, soya lecithin (E322) and MSG;
- many gluten-free convenience products (check labels).

Dairy foods and eggs make good protein replacements for vegetarians, but soya-intolerant vegans must seek expert advice. Grains, nuts, seeds, pulses, beans and avocados are the protein-rich foods to aim for. Also, look for 'soya free' on food labels.

Corn/maize

This is principally a Stateside problem, where corn is used and consumed in abundance. Products to avoid or look out for include:

- sweetcorn kernels and corn on the cob;
- corn flakes and other cereals;
- tortilla wraps and chips, tacos and other snacks;
- many ready meals, soups and sauces;
- corn meal and Italian polenta;
- low-gluten snacks and treats;
- some baking powders;
- any food label reading edible starch, food starch, modified starch, vegetable starch, cereal starch, glucose syrup (all may be corn or maize-derived), corn syrup, maltodextrin or dextrose (although these may have only traces of trigger proteins and will be safe for many).

Meats

Beef and pork appear to be the bigger villains in adults, although chicken is occasionally reported (particularly in children). Possible reactions include skin complaints such as urticaria and eczema. One unusual phenomenon sometimes encountered is beef intolerance in those suffering from CMPI, and chicken intolerance in those with egg intolerance, both possibly due to a cross-reaction between alike proteins.

Meat exclusion is not difficult, unless you are a devoted consumer, in which case lamb is often an ideal selection, as it appears to be tolerated by most. More exotic meats – such as venison or ostrich – are options but potentially laborious to source. A temporary pesco-vegetarian diet is a good move, as meat overconsumption could be the reason why the passionate carnivore develops an intolerance in the first place.

Excellent alternative iron-rich foods include shellfish, pulses, beans, seeds, chocolate and dried fruits.

Potato

Much-loved and heavily consumed in the UK, the humble spud is almost bound to be a likely candidate for food intolerance, such is the sense of satisfaction and comfort it conjures up. Who can resist the lure of a crisp, a chip or a baked potato fresh out of the oven and lavished with butter?

Providing you don't suffer cravings, eliminating potato is not hard. The obvious foods aside, you may find it as an added ingredient in some ready-meals, perhaps in the form of potato starch used as a thickener. Potato flour is often used in low-gluten foods, so coeliacs may have to look elsewhere for staples and treats.

Fish

You might expect fish to be a major culprit in immune-mediated food intolerance, given that it is a common guilty party in allergy – yet this does not seem to be the case, probably because most people's fish consumption is moderate.

The *food*SCAN only tests for tuna individually, with other fish grouped together in related combinations (such as crustaceans, molluscs and oily fish), so you may not have to eliminate all fish if you have a positive IgG outcome to one or more groups.

Blanket elimination, where necessary, will reduce your intake of the essential fatty acids for which seafood is celebrated, so ensure to eat a variety of nuts (walnuts, brazils) and seeds (pumpkin, sunflower) to compensate.

Fish is also an important source of iodine, vital for thyroid function. Sea vegetables, onions, pineapple and iodized salt are alternative sources.

Miscellaneous reactions

All foods containing protein – fruits and vegetables included – can produce an IgG-mediated reaction, but the following are alternative possible responses to the categories of food covered in this chapter, collected here for the mundane reason that they don't fit neatly elsewhere.

Tomatoes

A relatively new addition to the British diet, tomatoes are now found in a bounty of foods and dishes and are a firm national favourite. Adverse responses attributed to them include acid heartburn and gastric complaints. Tomatoes may also cause problems for those sensitive to glycoalkoloids (see Chapter 10) or MSG (Chapter 11).

Avoidance may not be easy, particularly if you follow a continental diet – watch out for all pasta sauces, chillies, pizzas, curries, condiments, concentrates, baked beans and soups, as well as any other prepared foods which are red, as tomatoes are often added to impart colour not taste.

You are unlikely to compromise your nutrition by having to omit tomatoes. However, they are the richest source of a red pigment called lycopene, which has generated considerable excitement among researchers for its superior antioxidant properties. Other, more moderate sources are watermelon, pink grapefruit and guava (but not berries, currants, grapes, cherries or plums).

Fats and oils

Digestive disruption is the principal symptom here. Gastric upset, nausea or vomiting after a fatty meal is not uncommon, and serves as a salutary warning to take it easier next time. Lower digestive malaise might imply that the body is mildly deficient in the bile or enzymes required to comprehensively digest fats. If undigested fats pass through to the colon a type of pale and fatty diarrhoea called steatorrhoea results.

Foods such as fatty meat, greasy chips and vegetable oils (and eggs and rich cheeses) are the typical bad guys when eaten in excess, but see your doctor if you experience chronic steatorrhoea as you may have an undiagnosed liver problem. Infrequent and mild bouts usually respond to moderation of fat consumption.

Oranges (and other citrus fruits)

One of the most commonly implicated fruits in food intolerance, probably due to overconsumption. The popular tendency of drinking large quantities of orange juice is often problematic, as its acidic nature can not only cause heartburn and indigestion, but potentially interfere with digestion by diluting enzymes.

Oranges are also high in benzoic acid, which can trigger red rashes around the mouth, especially in children. These are not dangerous. Other fruits, such as cranberries, may effect similar symptoms.

Mushrooms

Trehalose is an unusual form of sugar unique to the fungi kingdom, and some people may have inadequate levels of the enzyme trehalase needed to digest it. As with lactose and sucrose intolerances, this is another disaccharidase deficiency, covered in earlier chapters. If you experience abdominal responses such as diarrhoea and bloating after a meal of mushrooms, you may be trehalase deficient. Symptoms are typically avoidable through a lowered intake.

10

Alcohol, caffeine and natural food chemicals

So far we have dealt with intolerances caused by nutrients – mainly proteins and carbohydrates – but up to 20% of us experience problems with non-nutrients in our diet. These come in three principal guises: chemicals taken recreationally (alcohol) or for their pharmacological – or drug-like – effects (caffeine); naturally occurring toxins; some food additives (all of which will be considered in the next chapter).

Responses tend to occur when the body is unable to adequately detoxify or eliminate such substances, often when confronted with excess amounts. Some of the mechanisms involved are not understood, although the immune system is not suspected. Almost all of us would react adversely to elevated levels of the chemicals commonly implicated in these intolerances, but such high doses can be difficult to obtain through diet.

However, some individuals experience unpleasant symptoms when exposed to moderate quantities. Many learn to avoid any offending foods – sometimes permanently, as is often necessary – but others may not know what these are. Elimination diets are not always successful, because the chemicals involved may be found in many foods. Reliable forms of testing are unavailable. What follows should help.

Alcohol

The arguments for and against alcohol are well-documented. On one hand, very moderate quantities can destress, offer cardiovascular benefits and lower cholesterol; on the other, to excess it can contribute to heart, liver and kidney disease, various cancers, mental illness and a host of other debilitating diseases.

As noted in Chapter 3, alcohol can contribute to LGS and therefore potentially encourage intolerance reactions. It also strains the digestive system in other ways, hindering enzyme production and the liver's detoxification processes, and depleting the body's reserves of certain vitamins and minerals.

In a sense, everybody is intolerant to alcohol, in that above a certain threshold, we all experience unpleasant symptoms of intoxication such as nausea, vomiting, vertigo and mental retardation.

Our tolerance levels fluctuate throughout our lives, depending largely on present levels of drinking. The more we drink, the more detoxification enzymes the body will produce to cope, and the more able we will be to tolerate high levels next time. If we drink small amounts or not at all, this enzyme production is scaled down, so much so that even a modest subsequent alcoholic intake can make us feel disproportionately tipsy.

Although tolerance levels vary, the underlying trend is of increasing intolerance as we age: a fact well-known to many in their thirties, fond of bemoaning the fact that they can't drink as they could in their twenties! These particular cases of alcohol intolerance are worth stressing:

- Some people suffer from a hereditary deficiency of the detoxification enzymes required to break alcohol down. This is common among those of an Asian or native American background, around half of whom are affected, and for whom even small quantities can bring on nausea, facial flushing, and other symptoms sometimes associated with heavier drinking and hangovers.
- Those with chronic allergic or intolerance conditions such as asthma, rhinitis, headaches and urticaria may find these exacerbated by alcohol. This is because it can cause vasodilatation – the opening up of blood vessels – and nasal blockage.
- Sufferers of ME, or chronic fatigue syndrome, are often extremely alcohol-intolerant.

Managing such a sensitivity may mean teetotalism. Alcoholic drinks aside, you might also wish to avoid chocolate liqueurs, dishes cooked in wine, Christmas puddings and other desserts laced with spirits, depending on your tolerance threshold.

Caffeine

The world's favourite stimulant 1,3,7-trimethylxanthine, to give it its full chemical name, is found in coffee, tea, some soft drinks (typically colas), chocolate and some medication. The bad press caffeine gets is not entirely justified – it is an excellent mental energizer and mood elevator; it can relieve asthmatic symptoms; it is a mild painkiller.

However, it is moderately addictive. Worse, it can induce a string of unpleasant short-term symptoms to those sensitive to it, including nausea, anxiety and agitation, tremors, mood swings, restlessness, heart arrhythmias, vertigo, headaches, sweats and sleep interruption. More menacing reactions of hyperventilation, panic attacks, migraines, vomiting, abdominal cramps and diarrhoea are not uncommon at higher doses. Long-term, it can underlie some cases of constipation. Caffeine also exacerbates LGS.

Those who can be more susceptible to caffeine sensitivity include: children, whose intake should be moderated; women expecting a child or on the Pill, who metabolise caffeine more slowly and so may experience symptoms for longer; newly reformed ex-tobacco users, who might find their sensitivity suddenly increased, since smokers break down caffeine more efficiently than non-smokers.

Because of its pharmacological effects, 'cold-turkey' withdrawal symptoms are also unpleasant, albeit short-lived, and include anxiety, irritability, sleepiness or fatigue, depression and headaches. If you suspect caffeine sensitivity, reduce your intake gradually. This approach may also enable you to identify a tolerable caffeine threshold.

Perversely, caffeine can have a sedative effect on a tiny minority of people. If you find the more coffee or tea you drink, the sleepier you get, 'inverse' caffeine sensitivity could be the reason. Again, try cutting back.

Coffee

Most who like to take caffeine like to take it in coffee. And if you want to curb your caffeine intake, you may find it hard to cut coffee out. Instant coffee packs a milder caffeine punch than ground. Semi-decaffeinated versions are making their way onto shelves; decaffeinated varieties have been there for decades, and are very low in caffeine, but not absolutely free of it.

Ersatz coffees made from such ingredients as chicory, dandelion root, acorns, figs and cereals are pale substitutes, though you may find them palatable.

Caffeine aside, coffee contains hundreds of other chemicals, a few of which may irritate the gastro-intestinal tract. Some find that coffee provokes indigestion and heartburn, probably because it can stimulate the secretion of gastric acids.

Others experience a laxative effect when drinking coffee, typically their first cup of the day. If you find this undesirable, be aware that it may not be the coffee that is to blame, but the *temperature* at which you drink it. Hot drinks can rapidly precipitate peristaltic waves in the gut, so you may want to take your mochas a little cooler.

Tea

Tea has less caffeine than coffee, so you may tolerate it better. Black, oolong, green and white tea all contain roughly similar levels, with black having the highest and white the lowest. A stronger brew gives a greater caffeine kick. Decaffeinated tea is widely available.

Redbush tea, which – unlike green or white tea – can be drunk with milk, is an excellent caffeine-free substitute, and is regularly consumed in its own right, especially in South Africa, where it is known by its Afrikaans name, *rooibosch*.

Fanciful concoctions of herbal, fruity or spicy 'teas' or tisanes are now endemic. Herbal tisanes such as camomile and mint are often taken as digestive aids, and are generally to be recommended over the fruity or spicy varieties, which in some may irritate the gut.

Soft drinks

Decaffeinated colas are options, but if you can avoid carbonated beverages entirely you will be doing your body a favour, as they have nothing to recommend them from a nutritional perspective.

Chocolate

All real chocolate is made from the cocoa bean, which is lower in caffeine than the coffee bean, but higher in theobromine, a related chemical, which may also affect some individuals. Dark chocolate contains more caffeine than milk. Paradoxically, dark may be a wiser choice if you are looking to lower your intake, since a couple of squares, eaten slowly, can satisfy a chocolate craving more readily than a huge bar of milk chocolate, which may contain a greater total caffeine content. Migraine sufferers beware, however.

White chocolate has negligible or no caffeine. Carob is an unconvincing no-caffeine substitute for chocolate, but fares better in cooking.

Painkillers

Some painkilling or cold and flu medications contain added caffeine, typically the stronger-acting versions often labelled 'extra'. A tablet can contain as much as 65mg, equivalent to a cup of instant coffee. If it isn't specified in the ingredients, the medicine should be free of caffeine.

Amines

The amines are a class of highly active chemicals, naturally present in a wide range of foods and essential to many of the body's living processes, especially those involving the blood, central nervous system and brain.

However, many amines are vasoactive, meaning they dilate or contract blood vessels and affect blood pressure. These so-called vasoamines, in large amounts, or even modest amounts in sensitive individuals, can cause a number of allergy-like symptoms, including urticaria, angioedema, flushing, heart arrhythmias, wheezing, nausea, cramps, diarrhoea, and also headaches and migraines – the two reactions the amines are perhaps most notorious for.

Due to the sometimes rapid onset of symptoms, and the similarity between symptoms of amine intolerances and IgE-mediated allergies – in which the body rapidly releases stores of the amine histamine – the conditions can sometimes be confused.

Histamine is found in strongly flavoured foods such as mature cheese (blue, Parmesan, Roquefort), red wines, yeast-based spreads, European sausages and salamis, tuna and mackerel. The level of histamine in fish can rise alarmingly through bacterial action when it is not stored at cool temperatures. Cooking will not deactivate the histamine, which imparts a metallic, peppery taste to the fish.

Foods rich in *tyramine* include strong, mature cheeses such as Camembert, Stilton and Cheddar, some red wines such as Chianti, pickled herrings, liver pâtés, spicy continental sausages, fermented soya products such as soy sauce and bean curd, yeast extracts, sauerkraut and oranges.

Serotonin is typically found in fruits, principally banana, pineapple, plums, kiwi, tomato and avocado, but also chocolate, wines and some fish.

Phenylethylamine is present in chocolate, red wine, rich mature cheeses, continental sausages and pickled foods.

Foods containing *dopamine* include banana and avocado.

If you suspect you react to certain levels of amine, you can experiment with modifying your diet to see whether your symptoms subside or disappear. Instead of rich, mature cheeses, try milder cheeses such as Mozzarella, cottage cheese or cream cheese, which are considerably lower in or free of amines. White wine is much less amine rich than red wine. Most fish are low in tyramine, but white fish are also low in histamine. Carob is free from both tyramine and phenylethylamine. In general, aim for unfermented, unmatured or not-overripe foods, which tend to be lower in the vasoamines.

Salicylates

These are a class of naturally occurring, aspirin-like chemicals which can effect intolerance reactions – typically in those sensitive to aspirin itself, which is usually experienced as indigestion or gastric or abdominal pain. In such cases, dietary salicylate can trigger allergy-like symptoms such as urticaria and angioedema, wheezing and asthma, flushing and rhinitis, as well as some digestive upsets.

Foods rich in salicylates include most fruits (especially berries, oranges, melons), some vegetables (cucumbers, olives), strong herbs and spices (such as curry, rosemary, paprika, thyme), honey, nuts and tea.

Foods low in salicylates include meats, fish, dairy products, cereals and grains, many vegetables, peeled pears and bananas.

Salicylate sensitivity is uncommon, but if you suspect it seek the advice of a dietitian as following a balanced low-salicylate diet can be tricky, especially for vegetarians or those with dairy or grain intolerances, not least because levels in fresh foods vary according to season and the soil in which they were grown.

Glycoalkoloids

The nightshade family of vegetables includes potatoes, tomatoes, peppers, chillies and aubergine. All contain varying levels of toxic, nicotine-like glycoalkaloids such as solanine (in potatoes) and tomatine (in tomatoes), while chillies also contain capsaicin, responsible for imparting their fiery taste, and a common intestinal irritant.

In practice, it is solanine in the humble spud which usually comes under suspicion. Present mostly just under the skin, solanine is lost when the potato is peeled. However, levels increase greatly when the potato has begun to green, sprout or been exposed to light or bruised – when it is generally advisable not to consume it.

Most of us can easily detoxify the glycoalkaloids in a typical portion of nightshade vegetables without any adverse side-effects whatsoever. A few, however, may experience general unwellness and unpleasant gastro-intestinal symptoms. If you suspect this sensitivity, it may be worth eliminating all nightshades, then reintroducing them gradually one at a time, potatoes last, to see whether you can identify one or more culprits.

The nightshades have also earned an unproven reputation for worsening arthritic pain. If you suffer, a six-month restriction can be attempted.

Remember to replace excluded vegetables with a wide range of others; sweet potatoes and yams are tubers unrelated to potatoes, so are permitted. If you eat a typically Mediterranean, Middle Eastern or Indian diet, consult a dietitian if you wish to exclude nightshades for an extended trial period.

Since tobacco is a nightshade, giving up smoking can certainly help.

Lectins

These are a class of proteins found in beans, peas, peanuts and lentils. Most are harmless. But in some beans, particularly kidney beans, the lectins can be more problematic. Normally, these are destroyed by soaking and cooking, but in individuals sensitive to lectins or if cooking hasn't been thorough enough, unpleasant digestive reactions akin to those of food poisoning – such as nausea, abdominal pain, diarrhoea, vomiting – can result.

Oxalates

These chemicals are found principally in spinach, rhubarb, Swiss chard and beetroot. In a tiny minority, they can irritate the lining of the gut and precipitate digestive upsets such as nausea, pain and diarrhoea.

Cyanogens

These are chemicals found in the pips and stones of most fruits, as well as in almonds, sorghum, cassava and lima beans. When eaten the cyanogens release toxic cyanides, the compounds which give almonds and marzipan their characteristic aroma. Those highly sensitive to cyanides can experience unpleasant digestive responses, such as nausea, vomiting and diarrhoea, as well as vertigo and headaches. There have been reports of severe illness through eating too many cyanogen-rich apricot kernels, for instance.

Isatins

The flesh of the rose stone fruits – apricots, cherries, peaches, greengages and plums – contain non-toxic substances called isatins. In humans (and other mammals), isatins act as laxatives which stimulate fluid secretion in the gut and prompt colonic contractions, encouraging rapid intestinal transit and bowel evacuation.

Some of us are particularly sensitive to isatins, and may experience inconvenient and uncomfortable large-intestinal contractions after consuming even very modest quantities of the rose stone fruits (or other fruits such as figs and dates, in which isatins may also be found).

Since isatins are soluble, rose stone fruit juices retain their laxative properties, a fact which probably accounts for prune juice's peerless bowel-emptying capability.

11

Food additives

Without food additives, we would find it impossible to eat the rich and varied diet of convenient and always available foods to which most of us in the western world have become accustomed. Additives colour, flavour, preserve, bulk, thicken, emulsify and stabilize. Many products we take for granted would not exist without them.

An additive is given an E-number when it has been evaluated and passed as safe by the European Community Scientific Committee on Food, subject to regulatory controls. For instance, many additives carry maximum specified levels of use over which manufacturers cannot go, and more stringent regulations apply to additives in food for babies and toddlers.

E-numbers are much maligned, not always deservedly so. Most additives are safe for most people. Indeed many are naturally occurring – E300, ascorbic acid, is merely vitamin C. That said, human beings were not designed to deal with chemicals added to their foods, so it is not surprising a number of us react adversely to some.

Children are especially susceptible. The Hyperactive Children's Support Group recommend a number of those mentioned below, mainly the colours, be excluded from kids' diets. Research is ongoing in this area, and the safety or unsafety of particular additives is regularly hotly debated and questioned among scientists, nutritionists and parents. Keeping a rigorous food diary on behalf of a child can help identify any possible culprits, but careful monitoring is required. Diagnosis is difficult because there are no tests for such intolerances, and one additive is rarely consumed in the absence of all others.

Considered here are just some of those most often implicated in food sensitivities. Not all of the reactions have been validated; in many cases there is anecdotal evidence only and the reported reactions disputed.

Colours (azo dyes/'coal tar' dyes)

The bright or bold azo colourings below have been variously implicated in a string of reactions, including wheezing, urticaria, angioedema, eczema, rhinitis, migraine, childhood hyperactivity, and in some cases digestive upsets, visual disturbances and other idiosyncratic responses. Asthma sufferers and those sensitive to aspirin or salicylates should be especially cautious, as they may be more vulnerable. All are listed with a few examples of the foods in which they may be found.

E102 Tartrazine. Soft drinks, cakes, confectionery, desserts, sauces, jellies as well as medicines.

E104 Quinoline yellow. Scotch eggs, haddock and ice lollies.

E107 Yellow 2G. Soft drinks.

E110 Sunset yellow. Sweets, desserts, jams, marzipan, jellies, squashes and canned drinks.

E120 Cochineal. Alcoholic drinks, desserts, sauces and confectionery.

E122 Carmoisine. Jellies, cakes and confectionery.

E123 Amaranth. Gravy granules, cake mixes, jellies and processed fruit products.

E124 Ponceau 4R. Soups, desserts, cake mixes and salamis.

E127 Erythrosine. Confectionery, desserts, cocktail cherries, tinned fruit, some fish products, salami and sausages, as well as dental disclosing tablets.

E128: Red 2G. Sausages, meat products and occasionally jams.

E129 Allura Red AC. Sweet snacks, condiments, biscuits and cakes.

E131 Patent Blue V. Scotch eggs.

E132 Indigo carmine. Confectionery and desserts.

E133 Brilliant Blue FCF. Sweets, drinks, tinned peas.

E142 Greens S. Tinned peas, mint sauces, confectionery, jellies and ice cream.

E151 Black PN. Confectionery, desserts, jams, sauces and savoury snacks.

E154 Brown FK. Snack foods, smoked fish and meats.

E155 Brown HT. Convenience chocolate products.

Preservatives

E200 and E202/E203: Sorbic acid and the sorbates

Used in jellies, cheeses, yoghurts, soups, pizzas, wines and many other products. May underlie some eczematic symptoms and urticaria in sensitive individuals.

E210 and E211–E219: Benzoic acid and the benzoates

Found in soft and alcoholic drinks, meats, pizzas, yoghurts, jam and fruit fillings, marinated fish, confectionery, cheeses and condiments. Have been implicated in hyperactivity, as well as wheezing, asthma, urticaria, angioedema and other allergy-like reactions, as well as digestive disturbances. Those sensitive to tartrazine or aspirin/salicylates may also have problems with the benzoates.

E220 and E221–E228: Sulphur dioxide and the sulphites

Widely used in such foods as cold meats, seafood, soft drinks, fruit juices, dried fruit, tinned vegetables and fruits, ready-prepared salads, pickles, desserts, confectionery, biscuits, wines, ciders and beers. Can trigger severe wheezing, chest-tightening or full-blown attacks in many asthmatics, as well as provoke headaches and migraines, urticaria and angioedema, and in exceptional cases anaphylaxis. In IBS sufferers, they may worsen digestive upsets.

E249–E252: Nitrites and nitrates

Used in many meats – such as bacon, sausages, ham and corned beef – as well as some cheeses, pâtés and pizzas. Can occasionally trigger vertigo, dermal symptoms, headaches and migraine, raised blood pressure; some reports of nausea, shortness of breath and hyperactivity.

E280 and E281–E283: Propionic acid and the propionates

Used principally in dairy products, and breads and flour products; implicated in headaches, migraines and other intolerance symptoms.

Antioxidants

E310–E312: Gallates

Antioxidants used in fats, oils, cereals, salad dressings and snack foods; reported to cause gastric irritation in some, and allergy-like reactions in asthmatics and salicylate sensitives.

E320/E321: BHA/BHT

Petroleum derivatives used in fats, oils and butters, chewing gum, stock cubes and instant potato products. Many cases of hyperactivity and allergy-like symptoms have been blamed on them.

Thickeners

E407: Carageenan

Seaweed-derived thickener which has lately been implicated in digestive disturbances and ulcerative colitis.

Sweeteners

E420–E422: Sorbitol, Mannitol and Glycerol

Natural bulk sweeteners used in an array of diet, 'low-carb' and diabetic foods. They are slowly and poorly absorbed, indigestible in the gut, and stimulate the bowel, all of which in some people gives rise to nausea, flatulence, abdominal disquiet, loose stools and diarrhoea, much in the same way as lactose does in those with lactase deficiency. Higher doses are more likely to have an effect.

E950–E952, E954: Acesulfame-K, Aspartame, Cyclamate and Saccharin

The four most common intense sweeteners used in foods, appearing in hundreds of diet foods, sugar-free confectionery, soft drinks, snacks and desserts. It is aspartame that has been the source of most concern – with reported reactions of migraines, hyperactivity, urticaria, digestive malaise and even mental disturbances – but, more rarely, the others have been claimed to cause allergy-like reactions too.

E965–E967: Maltitol, lactitol, xylitol

Like sorbitol, mannitol and glycerol (E420-E422), these are sugar alcohols used as bulk sweeteners, and may elicit similar intolerance reactions.

Flavour enhancers

E620, E621 and E622-E625: Glutamic acid, MSG and other glutamates

The most infamous of these is E621 or monosodium glutamate (MSG), which is widely used, especially in Chinese cuisine, to heighten taste. The range is found in other savoury meat products, soups, sauces, tinned foods, dressings, prepared frozen meals and 'low-salt' foods. Glutamate is also present, sometimes naturally, in rich cheeses (Parmesan, Rocquefort), crisps and savoury snacks, piquant sauces (Worcestershire, soya), stock cubes, yeast spreads, dried fruit, ripe tomatoes, mushrooms, peas, wines, ports and sherries.

A number of adverse effects have been catalogued, especially in asthma and allergy sufferers, including typical reactions of nausea, wheezing and tightness in the chest, rhinitis, flushing and burning and headache, but also dizziness, low blood pressure and confusion.

The symptoms are known collectively as 'Chinese Restaurant Syndrome', in reference to its chefs' generous use of MSG. But it is far from proven that glutamates, and not other components of MSG-rich foods, are causing the reactions.

E635: Disodium 5'-ribonucleotides

This is a mix of disodium guanylate (E627) and disodium inosinate (E631). Extremely itchy urticarial rashes, often delayed and chronic, have been attributed to them. Allergy and intolerance writer and campaigner Sue Dengate, of the Food Intolerance Network of Australia, has dubbed disodium 5'-ribonucleotides 'the new MSG' and the urticaria it purportedly induces 'Ribo-rash'.

12

Other adverse reactions to food

Intolerances and allergies apart, there are other adverse reactions to food worthy of consideration – the most important being aversions.

What is food aversion?

Food aversions take a number of forms. Some are irrelevant; others, serious. As with intolerances and allergies, the definitions and categorization of aversions are a little confused. In its most literal interpretation, a food aversion is nothing more than just that – an intense dislike of a food, generally for reasons of unpalatability. It can be a permanent condition – most of us hate, and will always hate, the taste of at least one food, such as sprouts or liver – but it can be temporary too.

Examples of transient aversion abound. For instance the sick patient, harbouring an infection, who refuses most or all food. Or the child who loathes cabbage but will probably grow out of it by his teens. Or even the expectant woman who develops a genuine distaste throughout her pregnancy for a previously consumed food, a manifestation which often co-exists with its opposite – the food *craving* – and usually vanishes in tandem with it post-partum.

All these responses are thought to be natural protective mechanisms: an ill body might simply be too concerned temporarily with fighting off a viral invasion to want to expend any of its energy stores on the process of digestion; bitter toxins in the cabbage might detrimentally affect a young digestive system too immature to detoxify them; while a newly unpalatable food in a mum-to-be may contain chemicals theoretically harmful to the unborn foetus.

Psychological rejection
All the above examples are purely physiological responses. But sometimes, a physiological response can feature psychological elements, sometimes predominantly.

One excellent example familiar to many is the transient aversion affecting a sizeable percentage of the population on 27 December each year, when confronted with the possibility of tucking into turkey for a third consecutive day. This may be a combination of a beneficial physiological response – the body's way of calling for an alternative collection of nutrients than those to which it has been recently, and abundantly, exposed – and a psychological one – that 'ugh-not-turkey-*again*' feeling.

Straightforward food rejection can be purely psychological, but non-problematic. Most of us make conscious, perfectly valid decisions to not eat certain foods on numerous personal grounds, for:

- health reasons (such as the refusal of junk food);
- weight control (calorific food);
- political reasons (food grown in 'boycotted' nations);
- ethical or moral reasons (meat and dairy rejection in veganism);
- cultural or religious beliefs (for example, a meat-free diet in Hinduism);
- fear (of eggs and beef during the salmonella and BSE crises, for instance).

These should not be thought of as food aversion, although aversion may develop from or be an element of some cases, as in the examples below.

Somatization

The link between mind and body is a strong one. That between the mind and the digestive system is particularly interactive. Think of that lurching hollow in your stomach when you are nervous, or of your loss of appetite when something has upset you emotionally.

Somatization is the manifestation of physical symptoms in the body due to entirely mental factors. Such responses may also be called *psychogenic* – they have their origins in and are induced by the mind. And food can be a catalyst.

An example is the animal-loving vegetarian who unwittingly eats meat disguised in an innocent-looking dish, and then reacts violently on learning of its inclusion. This is a powerful instance of somatization – the mind rejects the food, and the body follows suit by vomiting.

Inducing an unpleasant, transient psychogenic response to food is simple. Merely thinking about and concentrating on an image of a dish of tripe, for instance, is enough to make many feel nauseous; ditto an outlandish combination of two separately non-controversial foods – a bowl of muesli topped generously with tomato ketchup should do the trick, and may well put you off both for days.

Somatization disorders

Such one-off reactions as those outlined above do not normally present a problem; the foods are simply avoided on a day-to-day basis. But when the food is a common one, and the reasons nothing to do with personal choice or revulsion, the situation may be more unsettling.

A food-mediated somatization disorder can be diagnosed when a person becomes strongly and falsely convinced that a particular food makes them ill – in other words, they believe they are intolerant or allergic to it. If the patient knowingly eats the perceived offender, one or more of the symptoms typically associated with food intolerance may result. Yet if the food is disguised and then fed to the sufferer, or it is eaten unawares or accidentally, no adverse responses occur.

That this form of adverse reaction to food is psychologically based in no way diminishes its legitimacy. The response is as real in the sufferer as a purely physiological reaction to gluten is in the coeliac.

Only one food may be involved. Delusional wheat intolerance is the most common example – the grain's relentless media trashing probably being responsible for many cases. It is not hard to fall victim to it – eliminating or cutting down on wheat can make anybody feel better, but drawing a conclusion of wheat intolerance from that may be quite wrong.

Alarmingly, a simple psychogenic intolerance to one food can escalate into multiple aversions. Patients believing they are being made ill in this way may impose on themselves increasingly stringent dietary limitations by eliminating a succession of foods, each based on illogical, self-diagnosed conclusions formulated from subjective interpretations of new 'reactions'. A mistaken opinion from one or more fringe practitioners can redouble the conviction, and therefore the problem, or can be the cause of the aversion to begin with.

More vulnerable to somatization disorders are patients with IBS. This is perhaps to be expected in those with 'hyper-sensitive' guts, since the mind-body link in them may be more volatile. Tension and stress are far more likely to manifest in physical responses in sufferers than in non-sufferers, and because the nature of the condition means that symptoms sometimes fluctuate anarchically, IBS patients can be led to speculate more readily on – and then casually exclude – supposed dietary triggers.

Diagnosis

Allergy UK reports regular cases of severe somatization disorders – people whose lives are blighted by obsessional anxieties centred on food and who fundamentally believe they're being poisoned by their diet. It is a desperate situation for those suffering, one which re-emphasises the importance of a sensible approach to solving possible food sensitivities.

Ideally, a diagnosis of somatization disorder can only be made with any degree of confidence when all accepted forms of testing and exclusion diets described in Chapters 4 and 5 and for allergy have failed to demonstrate a physical disease or food sensitivity. If a doctor can find no obvious cause, an organ specialist no disease, and an allergist no allergy, then the onus may well fall on the dietitian to identify the problem.

Many dietitians will do their utmost to eliminate the possibility of food aversion before considering intolerance; a patternless, coming-and-going of symptoms may be one indication of it, but the skill of identification often comes with experience. In practice, somatization may only suggest itself when the exclusion phase of a strict elimination diet fails to bring an improvement.

A sympathetic approach is required from the patient's medical practitioners, several of whom might have a role to play in reaching a diagnosis. A doctor, for instance, may also need to consider a patient's background – a history of depression, say, can strengthen the case for somatization, as might a recent emotional upheaval.

Somatizing patients can be resistant to their diagnosis, blaming their healthcare providers for failing to find the 'real' cause. An experiment to 'prove' the psychogenic response may be attempted, usually taking the form of a double-blinded test, where the patient is fed disguised samples of supposed culprit foods and of innocent foods, while responses are monitored by a specialist also unaware of which foods are which.

If the absence of a reaction to a positive feed can be shown, this can go some way towards demonstrating the absence of a physical problem, but in practice the procedure is expensive, time-consuming, and often fails anyway – simply because the patient is wary and expectant of a reaction so suffers one after each sample.

In fairness, somatization can be overdiagnosed by some doctors faced with patients presenting non-specific symptoms. Equally, though, overzealous practitioners may be too keen to diagnose physiological food intolerance and miss or ignore a psychological aversion.

Treatment

Treatment is vital – and not only because of the threat of malnutrition and the misery inflicted on the sufferer and the sufferer's loved ones. Like all people, somatizers are truly ill from time to time, and there is a real danger when this happens of a doctor missing a serious physiological condition producing symptoms he mistakenly assumes to be psychosomatic.

Patients should be encouraged to eat a full and nutritious diet, on the basis that if a full diet makes the patient ill, and a limited diet also makes a patient ill, then the full diet is preferable from a nutritional standpoint.

Counselling is also to be recommended, although sufferers can feel affronted at the suggestion, and so this depends largely on their consent to treatment.

Food poisoning

This form of adverse reaction is unique in that it does not normally discriminate: anybody who consumes a food or drink contaminated with certain live pathogenic bacteria, viruses, parasites or powerful toxins is likely to suffer similar, strong reactions – normally vomiting, abdominal pain, violent diarrhoea and sometimes fever, excessive perspiration, muscular aches and exhaustion.

It is worth remembering that a bout of food poisoning or gastroenteritis can be a precursor to a food intolerance, so following a bland diet (water, rice, plain vegetables, bananas, for example) during and after the attack is advisable to give the gut ample time to recover from any inflammation or damage.

For further advice about food poisoning, including food safety and food hygiene, see www.foodlink.org.uk.

Food phobia

In exceptional cases, an individual may be truly phobic towards a certain food, and suffer symptoms of extreme anxiety, distress or terror towards it. The root cause can often be traced back to a traumatic childhood experience with which the patient associates the food – for instance, one of choking on baked beans. Some forms can be quite unique – a morbid fear of asparagus, due to its unorthodox shape and form, has been reported.

The National Phobics Society can advise (tel: 0870 770 0456; website: www.phobics-society.org.uk).

Food neophobia

This is a slight misnomer, not being a true phobia at all. It is the natural trepidation or suspicion with which many of us regard a new or exotic food, such as escargot, ostrich or even the now mainstream sushi.

Neophobia is thought to be a natural genetic throwback to our time as ancestral hunter-gatherers, when caution towards an unknown foodstuff was a necessary survivalist trait. Many of us will tentatively sample a tiny quantity of a new food, as our remote forefathers might have done, to see how it agrees with us. Often, we will find it palatable and, emboldened, consume more. Occasionally, we will reject it permanently.

It is particularly prevalent in children under ten, around three-quarters of which will occasionally refuse foods with which they are not familiar. Parents should avoid applying pressure. Seeing the family contentedly eating the food in question is usually enough motivation for children to try it when they are ready.

Food neophobia is usually a transient aversion, and is generally outgrown.

13
Living with food intolerance

Living on a restricted diet can be tough, particularly if you are required to remove more than one common food. There may be times when you feel poorly or 'grotty', especially during the early days. 'No pain, no gain' is a maxim overused in the sphere of health and fitness, but in this case it might fairly apply.

But that does not mean you cannot do it. Just the opposite, in fact. By being organized and committed about your wellbeing and recovery, by persevering with your dietitian's recommendations, and by making the most of all the information and support that is available, you will succeed.

Shopping

A natural concern is that you will have to radically alter your shopping routine, but in practice this is rarely the case. Most supermarkets now offer wide ranges of specialist-diet foods, and your local healthfood store is likely to be similarly well-stocked. Several mail-order suppliers have sprung up to meet increasing demands, as have 'free-from' food manufacturers specializing in niche ranges.

Labelling
Something you will have to be more conscientious about is reading labels. Bear these points in mind:

- Common ingredients can be camouflaged under unfamiliar names, such as caseinate (a milk protein) and ovalbumin (an egg protein).
- Check for hidden sugars in ready-meals by reading the nutritional details on the label. Carbohydrate content will be given, usually followed by an 'of which sugars' reading which gives the level of simple monosaccharide and disaccharide sugars in the food (lactose included).
- Look for confirmation of the absence or presence of potentially reactive foods. Such terms as 'free from dairy' or 'contains fish' are now standard. Many producers are also adopting icons such as a 'V' for vegan or vegetarian, and assorted 'No Wheat' signs.

- Remember that all vegetarian foods are by definition meat and fish-free and that all foods labelled vegan are additionally dairy-free and egg-free.
- So-called defensive labelling – 'may contain traces of peanut', for example – is being increasingly frowned upon by campaigners who see it is as confusing and frustrating to food sensitives. It is used by manufacturers as a pre-emptive disclaimer of liability in the remote event of a product being accidentally contaminated by an allergen and then consumed by someone prone to anaphylaxis. While generally of less concern to food intolerants, any 'may contain gluten/wheat' notice should be heeded by coeliacs.
- Do not be lulled into false security by a bright 'no artificial additives' label – a lot of additives, such as a number of sweeteners, are naturally occurring and will not be covered by such a disclaimer.
- Be equally alert around organic food. Organic does not imply 'additive free'. For instance, the vegetable dye annatto (E160b) is found in some traditionally coloured cheeses such as Double Gloucester and Red Leicester, certain moderated levels of sulphur dioxide (E220) are used to prevent oxidation and as a preservative in organic wines and ciders, while sodium nitrite (E250), potassium nitrate (E251) and sodium nitrate (E252) are all allowed in the curing of organic bacons and hams. Other permitted additives include calcium carbonate (E170), lecithin (E322) and carageenan (E407).
- Do not assume you will have to abandon all your most cherished treats. If labels on favourite foods carry ambiguous or generic terms such as 'starch' or 'vegetable oil' – which have several possible sources – do not reject the food without first contacting the manufacturer for clarification. If necessary, ask whether a free-from version or replacement product is available or can be recommended.

Cooking

Changes to your cooking routine depend so much on the nature of your intolerances and whether you normally cater solely for yourself, or have a partner or children to consider too, that it is difficult to give generalized advice. Whatever your circumstances, you will find your own way of adapting and managing.

If you are cooking for others, you may have to guard against absent-minded food sampling and learn to ignore the cravings that the aromas will undoubtedly spark off. Issues of cross-contamination in the kitchen are usually only of significance to coeliacs, who should keep separate bread bins, bread boards and spreads, for example – a toast crumb left behind in the butter tray can be enough to activate an adverse response.

There will be occasions when you and your family can eat the same meals. However, if your diet eliminates numerous staples, regularly imposing similar restrictions on children is not only unfair, but can affect their nutrition too.

Experiment with new ingredients, so you avoid coming to rely on a favourite 'replacement' food. Recipe ideas abound on the internet – enter something like 'egg free cooking' into a decent search engine.

Dozens of cookery books devoted to restricted diets are available too. Try Barbara Cousins' *Cooking Without* books or any by Antoinette Savill. Endeavour to find one written with your sensitivity in mind – some 'all-purpose' free-from cookbooks tend to exclude most reactive foods from most recipes, including those to which you may not be intolerant.

If you are concerned about nutrient intake, supplementation may be advised. Speak to your dietitian or doctor. Do not supplement without professional input. Equally, never skip meals, or assume you can compensate for them with vitamin pills.

'Cheating'

'Just a little mouthful won't hurt,' says a devillish voice in your head. But how to respond? Because you will probably feel healthier, the temptation to sneak a bite of a much-missed food may be a constant presence. Whether or not this will harm you depends on how long you have been following your diet and which intolerance you have.

If you are lactase deficient, for instance, you might be able to get away with a spoonful of ice cream. Or you might not, and instead suffer the runs within the hour.

If you have a suspected IgG-mediated intolerance, you should resist temptation. Cheating in this instance is effectively reintroducing the food prematurely, before your dietitian's or nutritionist's recommended elimination time. Potentially, this can tax your immune system unnecessarily and undo a lot of the good work you have done so far. Is it *really* worth it?

And if you are a coeliac, cheating is plain dangerous. Take your frustration out on a punchbag, scream at the top of your voice, console yourself with a gluten-free treat – then feed that chunk of French bread to the ducks instead.

Eating away from home

This is gradually becoming less of a problem as society grows increasingly mindful of food intolerance – but you still have to exercise care. Friends may not understand your situation, and it is up to you to impress upon them the importance of their not feeding you gluten, for instance, when you are asked to dinner. If you sense nervousness, offer to help with the cooking, to bring your own ingredients or food, or ask them to yours instead. If you sense deep scepticism, decline the invite.

Eating out presents bigger stumbling blocks. Food served at cafés, sandwich shops and snack bars, for instance, may not have been made on site and rarely carries labelling. Polite enquiries of staff might not yield trustworthy information. If in doubt, rule it out.

Restaurants are safer bets. Waiters and chefs are now accustomed to specific dietary needs. Here are some tips: call the restaurant in advance to enquire whether it can cater for you; be explicit about your requirements and don't be shy of articulating the implications of any contamination; ask the waiter or a chef to recommend a suitable dish for you; send back a meal which you suspect has not been prepared according to your request; double-check with the waiter before you tuck in; make a point at the end of the meal of thanking staff personally for serving and catering for you.

The websites www.harid.co.uk and www.foodfreefrom.co.uk offer searchable directories of recommended eateries.

Holidays and travel

This need not be a problem. There are many intolerance-friendly guesthouses and hotels, both in the UK and abroad, which will welcome you. Look for some on the two websites above, or else try your luck on a search engine.

When planning to go abroad, choose countries whose cuisines are unlikely to trouble you. For instance, Asian destinations are usually suited to wheat and dairy intolerants, but not ideal for those sensitive to rice or soya.

Foods Matter magazine can provide thorough and invaluable 'free-from' ingredient lists translated into six European languages.

Allergy UK have a factsheet on airline travel and also offer a translation card service.

Depression

Low moments will come and go. One helpful tactic is to think of your maintenance diet in terms of 'choice' – rather than viewing it as something which has been forced upon you. This is an effective form of self-empowerment. Feeling excluded from everyday social experiences – not being able to share that 24-inch pizza with your family, for example – is a common problem. As is missing favourite foods.

Stay positive. Surround yourself with encouraging people. Treat yourself in any way you can, even with a box of chocolates occasionally – dairy-free if necessary. Remind yourself that you are 'choosing' to do this, and that you are 'choosing' to get well. And if you need to, call a support line and talk to someone.

Negative attitudes

Although attitudes are changing, sympathy and understanding are sentiments not yet universally expressed towards food intolerants. Inevitably, some people will see you as a 'fussy' eater; others will unfairly tar your condition with the 'fad diet' brush. This can be upsetting when people to whom you are close are the perpetrators.

It is important to challenge these views and impress the gravity of your condition, not only for your own pride and confidence but also to foster a wider understanding of food sensitivities. Do not say 'I don't eat wheat', say 'I *can't* eat wheat', and add 'for medical reasons' if you have to. Be firm, be polite, be unrepentant. Vegans, Jews and diabetics, to name but three groups, do not – and should not – apologize for their dietary restrictions, and neither should you. Why on earth should you feel awkward about what does and does not enter your body?

Stress

Do not underestimate how seriously this can shackle your recovery. Your diet is controllable. Your stress levels may be largely *un*controllable. Because of this, most food intolerants would prefer it if their problems were caused exclusively by food, yet evidence suggests that stress is often heavily implicated. This is especially true of IBS sufferers.

If you do not have the time or energy to nourish yourself properly, to sit down, relax and enjoy your own home-cooked meals – then you are probably too busy, and probably too stressed. And if you are too stressed, then you are hindering your chances of getting well.

It is beyond the scope of this book to offer suggestions about 'down-scaling' or work/life balance, but do at least ask yourself honestly whether your level of suffering is ultimately a price worth paying to maintain your lifestyle. If you find yourself in an interminable tunnel of stress, with no sign of light at the end, consider making some major changes to how you live.

Psychotherapy

This is not as extreme as it may sound. Counselling as part of stress management can help with a breadth of problems. Psychologically, merely getting feelings off your chest can bust anxiety.

More advanced forms of treatments may also be of value. Hypnotherapy is one option; while cognitive behaviour therapy (CBT) challenges the way you think, feel and how you respond to those sentiments. It can help eliminate false ideas and negative thoughts ('I'll never get better; I may as well eat what I like') which can overwhelm you and impede recovery.

Controlled trials employing both CBT and hypnotherapy on IBS sufferers have demonstrated significant improvements in both physiological and psychological symptoms.

Speak to your doctor, or contact the British Association of Behavioural and Cognitive Psychotherapies (01254 875277; www.babcp.com).

Complementary therapies

Please choose wisely. Please do not spend vast sums of money. Please do not undergo any obviously suspect therapy. Simple, purely therapeutic treatments such as massage and meditation undoubtedly counter stress, and may well justify and reward your time and investment. But for many, the home therapy option is far cheaper and more reliable – a steaming hot bath, some aromatherapy massage oils, an abundance of candles, and an ambient soundtrack of gentle music.

Reintroduction . . . and recovery

Permanent exclusions excepted, the time will come when you can reintroduce those foods to which you once reacted or tested positive. If you are being treated via a dietitian, he will advise you. If you have taken the *food*SCAN, you will have received recommendations from **YORK**TEST, but you can make use of the telephone support available to you if you need it.

In the latter case, foods should be reintroduced after three months, six months, nine months or twelve months, depending on the quantity of IgG antibodies to individual foods originally found in your blood sample. The more there were, the longer your system needs to remove them, and the longer you will have had to exclude the food.

To test dairy, **YORK**TEST advise eating a portion of yoghurt first (although evaporated milk is also a good option); with wheat, a 100% wholewheat cereal, and with egg, a cooked yolk. Remember to monitor any reactions in a food diary.

You might also like to have someone with you when you reintroduce. Keep any medication – such as an asthma inhaler – close at hand too, in the very unlikely event of an alarming response. If you do have one, you will probably have to exclude the food for another period of, on average, six months.

In the absence of symptoms, other related foods (breads, wholemilks, etc.) can then be tried, and later incorporated into your diet on a four-day rotation plan. Providing you stay healthy, this can later be increased to three days, and then more frequently if you wish and can tolerate it – but you must guard against slipping back into any old habits of overconsumption.

If you are reintroducing more than one food, only move onto subsequent foods after a week or so, once previous ones have been comfortably reincorporated.

Coeliac disease

You will be advised and monitored closely during the first and perhaps second years after a coeliac diagnosis to ensure your health is improving and your gut recovering through ongoing gluten exclusion. A second 'check-up' biopsy may be recommended.

14

Staying well

Most people are aware of the sensible guidelines regarding eating lots of fruit and vegetables, taking exercise and quitting smoking. But what this chapter aims to offer you are some additional health tips you may not have considered before, specifically aimed at preventing new or former food intolerances and the symptoms associated with them.

Healthy Eating

Food intolerance is generally caused by some failure or breakdown of the digestive process, so any strategy to prevent it ought to be principally concerned with ideas of good eating practice.

Ask your body what it wants you to eat

Take your time. Think carefully. Do not just mindlessly finish off whatever is in the fridge or yesterday's leftovers.

Have a place to eat

If you eat where you watch television, or you eat where you work, or – worse – you eat on the move, you fail to send your body the key message that you have decided to rest, relax and concentrate on nothing but nutrition and digestion for an hour. Move away from the sofa or desk and find somewhere to sit where you can focus on eating. And nothing else.

Cook it, savour it

One of the tragedies of the grab-a-sandwich, take-away, ready-meal culture we live in is that many have abandoned the enjoyment and benefits of meal preparation. Cooking is important – it's soothing, grounding and relaxes you before you eat. Aromas are key too – they stimulate your digestive system to ready itself for what it is about to receive. Eating fast food robs your body of all that. It gives it not only what it may not want, but also what it is not prepared for.

Have fewer ingredients in your meal

Eat larger portions of fewer foods at one sitting, rather than smaller portions of more foods. The greater number of foods you eat, the more digestive enzymes your body will need to produce, and the harder it will have to work – not always a good thing. The 'meat and two veg' approach may be a sound tradition. But remember to always choose different vegetables every day, and to rotate the meats with fish, eggs and grains.

Eat as nature intended

Apples grow on trees. Apple pies do not. Apples are whole foods. Apple juice is merely apples stripped of their fibre – fibre required by the body to facilitate the fruit's digestion. Go for the natural whole food when you can.

Liberate your digestive system

Do not slouch when you eat. Keeping your back straight keeps your stomach in an optimal position. Equally, avoid wearing tight clothing, which also impedes the digestive organs.

Take your time

Chew slowly and thoroughly. The more food is physically broken down, the more efficiently you will digest it. The lengthier contact food has with the amylase in your saliva, the more effective the process of starch digestion will be. Both relieve some of the strain on your body of carrying out more advanced digestive processes. Eat in company – you are less likely to wolf your food down.

Do not overeat

Eating heavily in one sitting strains the digestive system. And if it cannot produce enough enzymes to cope, more undigested food molecules will be absorbed into your system, increasing the likelihood of a reaction. Stop eating when your body tells you it is no longer hungry. You can always eat a little more later.

Do not force food onto your body

Making unreasonable demands on your digestive system is a sure-fire way to gastro-intestinal dissent. Avoid 'finishing off' food fast approaching its use-by date if your body does not want it; throw it out if you have to. Don't accept coffee and biscuits when visiting a friend if your body says no, even if your friend protests. Be polite, but firm. It is not rude to refuse.

Get antioxidizing

Antioxidants are naturally occurring chemicals which attack oxidants – unstable substances manufactured by the body as normal by-products of metabolic processes. Vitamin C and quercetin are two fine specimens of antioxidant. Vitamin C is thought to benefit a number of digestive processes, and deficiency has been associated with food intolerance. Quercetin, meanwhile, is a powerful bioflavonoid known for its internally healing and antiseptic qualities on the gut. You will find both in apples and onions.

Drink less when you eat

Too much liquid when you eat, especially acidic ones like juices and wines, can dilute gastric fluids and enzymes, hampering digestion.

Eat with the seasons

Not only does seasonal produce taste really good, it is likely to be better for you, as it will have been grown under less artificial conditions, and be richer in nutrients. This practice is a natural way to guard against eating a particular fruit or vegetable all year round, something likely to protect you from developing an intolerance towards it. And who wants strawberries in winter anyway?

Rotate your carbs

Rice one day, wheat the next, potatoes the next, millet the next – that kind of thing.

Eat what your ancestors ate

Following a diet typical of your ethnic background could be a good move, as you are likely to have inherited the appropriate selection of enzymes to digest it. Some westerners simply cannot comfortably handle the spicy, exotic foods of East Asia; just as those from East Asia cannot tolerate a western diet featuring dairy products and alcohol.

Ditch the fad diets

They meddle with your biology, as any dietitian will tell you. And any programme which encourages you to eat a large volume of a particular food – be it grapefruit or cabbage soup, for instance – should be avoided for a number of reasons, not least because of the risk of becoming intolerant to that food.

Trash the gum

Just after a meal is okay, but chewing gum at other times merely gets digestive juices flowing and the body working for no good reason. There is no food for the enzymes to digest – a waste of vital body fluids and deeply confusing to your system.

Stay put when you stop

Don't rush back to work or into a physical activity when you finish eating – give your body some time to devote its energies to digestion.

Healthy Living

Staying intolerance-free isn't solely a matter of healthy eating, however . . .

Reduce your chemical exposure

Do you jog during rush hour? Are you liberal in your use of household air fresheners and furniture polishes? Do you use cosmetics every day?

The environment is becoming ever more polluted, something which threatens us all, not only asthmatics. Meanwhile, according to Allergy UK, 'the increased use of chemicals both in cleaning and sweetening our homes, offices and schools are adding to the load that our systems are having to fight to stay healthy'.

Consider going for your run when traffic fumes are at their lowest, very early or late in the day, or at least in the mid-day hours. Open windows to freshen the atmosphere at home and wipe tabletops with nothing more than a damp cloth. Choose green, natural or organic cosmetics and toiletries.

Go when you have to go

Some people don't like to go in an unfamiliar toilet, such as the one at work. Others deem it an unforgivable insult to go at a friend's house. When your bowels are signalling to you that they would like to open, be kind to them and obey. Holding on increases the likelihood of a painful motion when you eventually do go, and encourages your body to reabsorb toxins which it needs to eliminate in your stool. And that can tax your liver unnecessarily. And give you a headache, tire you, or adversely effect the rest of your digestive system. And make your breath smell.

Make yourself at home in the company loo. And as far as your friend is concerned, you have been gone a while because you were admiring the lovely tiles.

Keep stress down

Nip it in the bud before it gets too much – for an abundance of reasons. To pick one at random: stress interferes with the production of sIgA, the antibody which lines the gut mucosa and targets any potentially reactive undigested proteins before they get the chance to irritate your bowel lining or enter your system.

The three best stress-busters are known to be laughter, exercise/getting away from it all and sex. Do whatever it takes – watch back-to-back videos of your favourite comedy, take a long stroll in the woods, make love with your partner.

If only these were the cures for everything.

Conclusion

So what of the future? Will we one day be able to pop some magic pill to banish our intolerances, and spare ourselves the sometimes wearisome process of curative dietary restrictions? It is unlikely. As we have seen, food intolerance is too protean and unpredictable, and varies too much from person to person. More research is undoubtedly required, as is investment in the management and prevention of intolerance, as is greater education and awareness. But there appears to be cause for optimism.

GM food

Whatever your views on this controversial topic, genetic modification of foods offers extraordinary possibilities. So-called allergy-free GM nuts were successfully produced in the late 1990s, and in 2002 scientists in Hawaii grew non-allergenic soya beans. Do not be surprised if you soon start to hear murmurings about low-gluten wheat grains and caffeine-free coffee too.

However, these fantastical developments may have unwanted side-effects. Removing, deactivating or otherwise altering trigger proteins or chemicals could, in theory, create unforseen new intolerance or allergy problems. So, GM solutions to food sensitivities may be some time off yet.

Improved labelling

Under European law, labelling is becoming more stringent. For example, the EU Allergens Directive requires all manufacturers in member countries to alert the consumer to any use of the most common reactive ingredients in their food products, namely: celery, eggs, fish, gluten, milk, mustard, peanuts, sesame, shellfish, soya, sulphur compounds (above concentrations of 10mg/kg or 10mg/litre) and tree nuts.

While this is a positive move, there is concern that some non-specialist manufacturers may be tempted to adopt excessive and unnecessary 'free-from' labelling tactics in an attempt to capture a share of the expanding special-diet market.

Research and healthcare provision

Many organizations are pushing forward on these long-neglected areas. Only two initiatives are briefly considered here.

The National Allergy Strategy Group, an umbrella alliance which includes Allergy UK and Action Against Allergy, is aiming to 'influence the development of allergy services by action through professional, political, public and patient interest channels'. Healthcare education, awareness programmes and governmental lobbying are included on its estimable manifesto. And while geared more towards allergy, sufferers of food intolerance will surely benefit from the NASG's work.

Meanwhile, the Food Standards Agency has set up a Working Group on Food Additives and Behaviour in Children to examine the links between E numbers and such problem issues as infant hyperactivity.

There is plenty of similar research, all of it driven by the aim of bridging the gaps in our understanding of food intolerance. Hopefully, that is something we will soon achieve.

Useful addresses

Many of the bodies and sources of information included here use alternative definitions and classifications of food sensitivities to those adopted in this book. Readers are advised to familiarise themselves with the conventions and categorisations being assumed when accepting advice from other organisations or healthcare professionals.

Organizations

Allergy UK
3 White Oak Square, London Road, Swanley, Kent BR8 7AG
Switchboard/Chemical Sensitivity Helpline: 01322 619898
Allergy Helpline: 01322 619864
Website: www.allergyuk.org or www.allergyfoundation.com

Action Against Allergy
PO Box 278, Twickenham, Middlesex, TW1 4QB
Tel: 020 8892 2711
E-mail: aaa@actionagainstallergy.co.uk
Website: www.actionagainstallergy.co.uk

YORKTEST Laboratories Ltd
York Science Park, York YO10 5DQ
Freephone and support line (UK only): 0800 074 6185
Tel: 01904 410410
Email: clientsupport@yorktest.com
Website: www.yorktest.com
For comprehensive ELISA IgG food testing, support literature and follow-up nutritional advice and information. The website links to branches in USA, Ireland, Australia, Germany, Austria, Italy, Greece and the UAE.

Coeliac UK
PO Box 220, High Wycombe, Buckinghamshire, HP11 2HY.
Tel: 01494 437278 or 0870 444 8804
Website: www.coeliac.co.uk

The IBS Network
Northern General Hospital, Sheffield S5 7AU
Telephone: 0114 261 1531
IBS Helpline: 01543 492192
Email: info@ibsnetwork.org
Website: www.ibsnetwork.org.uk

Useful websites

www.allallergy.net
Perhaps the only website you need: a comprehensive gateway to literally thousands of allergy- and intolerance-related organizations, events, publications and products worldwide.

www.allergy-network.co.uk and www.allergy-clinic.co.uk
Superlative sites, teeming with information on intolerance and allergy, written by Dr Adrian Morris of the Surrey Allergy Clinic.

www.allergysa.org
Excellent resource from the Allergy Society of South Africa.

www.asthma.org.uk
Asthma UK.

www.candida-society.org
Website of the National Candida Society.

www.celiac.com
American-based resource for coeliacs and wheat intolerants.

www.corecharity.org.uk
Core (formerly The Digestive Disorders Foundation).

www.eatwell.gov.uk
Foods Standard Agency-run site with advice on food safety, food labelling and more.

www.eczema.org
The National Eczema Society.

www.faia.org.uk
Site of the Food Additives and Ingredients Association.

www.fedupwithfoodadditives.info

Extremely useful website from Sue Dengate of the Food Intolerance Network of Australia.

www.foodandmood.org
Website of the Food and Mood Project, exploring the relationship between 'what you eat and how you feel'.

www.foodintol.com
Excellent Australian website offering support and information to sufferers of all food sensitivities.

www.fdf.org.uk
The Food and Drink Federation's website, with links to sister sites devoted to food safety and hygiene, 'food fitness', and 'food future', which covers GM food issues.

www.foodcanmakeyouill.co.uk
Useful website from writer and researcher Sharla Race.

www.foodyoucaneat.com
Links, news and forums aimed at US-based sensitives.

www.hacsg.org.uk
The Hyperactive Children's Support Group.

www.lactose.co.uk
Superior source of information for those with lactose intolerance, milk sensitivities, IBS and other related conditions.

www.migraine.org.uk
The Migraine Action Association.

www.nacc.org.uk
National Association for Colitis and Crohn's Disease (NACC).

www.noarthritis.com
Website of the US-based Arthritis Nightshades Research Foundation.

www.soilassociation.org
The Soil Association's website, with information on organic food, suppliers and organizations.

www.ukfibromyalgia.com

Information resource for sufferers of FM or FMS.

www.vegansociety.com
Food and nutritional advice from the Vegan Society on meat, fish, dairy and egg-free eating.

www.vegsoc.org
Website of the Vegetarian Society, with advice on meat- and fish-free eating.

www.worldallergy.org
Website of the World Allergy Organization.

Online discussion groups

Web-based public discussion forums can offer terrific support and information, although some can be unruly at times. Advice is generally well meant, but it can never replace authoritative medical opinion. Here are just two, but you can find dozens of others via some of the websites listed above, or by entering terms such as 'food intolerance discussion' or 'online allergy forum' into a good search engine.

www.alt.support.food-allergies
A lively forum covering intolerance as well as allergies. Find it through groups.google.com/

www.health.groups.yahoo.com/group/FCMYI/
'Food Can Make You Ill' – a group open to those suffering from any food sensitivity, their relatives, and interested healthcare professionals.

Retailers and manufacturers

Supermarkets
Most major supermarkets offer wide ranges of special-diet foods, leaflets, and web information.
Asda 0500 100055; www.asda.co.uk
Budgens 0800 526 002; www.budgens.co.uk
Co-op 0800 068 6727; www.co-op.co.uk.
Iceland 01244 842842; www.iceland.co.uk
Kwik Save 0117 935 6669; www.kwiksave.co.uk

Marks and Spencer 0845 302 1234; www.marksandspencer.com
Morrisons 01924 870000; www.morereasons.co.uk
Safeway 01622 712987; www.safeway.co.uk
J Sainsbury 0800 636262; www.sainsbury.co.uk
Somerfield 0117 935 6669; www.somerfield.co.uk
Tesco 0800 505555; www.tesco.com
Waitrose 0800 188884; www.waitrose.com

Health food stores

Likely to be good sources of products free from gluten, wheat, milk, eggs, soya, sugar, caffeine and artificial chemicals, as well as digestive enzyme supplements.

Holland and Barrett 0870 606 6605; www.hollandandbarrett.co.uk.
GNC 0845 601 3248; www.gnc.co.uk.

Mail order and on-line suppliers

Allergy Free Direct 01288 356396; www.allergyfreedirect.com. *A wide range of specialist foods.*
Dietary Needs Direct 01527 579086; www.dietaryneedsdirect.co.uk. *Mainly products free from gluten and casein.*
Gluten Free Foods Direct 01757 630725; www.glutenfreefoodsdirect.co.uk. *Gluten- and wheat-free foods.*
GoodnessDirect 0871 871 6611; www.goodnessdirect.co.uk. *Three thousand products free from wheat, gluten, dairy, egg, yeast and caffeine.*

'Free-from' food companies

Arla Foods 0113 382 7000; www.lactolite.co.uk. *Low-lactose milk.*
Bakers Delight 0845 120 0038; www.bakers-delight.co.uk. *Wheat- and gluten-free bread, cakes, pies and puddings.*
D&D 024 7637 0909; www.d-dchocolates.com. *Carob and dairy-free chocolate products, including seasonal lines.*
Delamere Dairy 01565 750528; www.delameredairy.co.uk. *Goats' milk products.*
Doves Farm 01488 684880; www.dovesfarm.co.uk. *Gluten-free flours, biscuits and cereals.*
Dietary Specials 07041 544044; www.nutritionpoint.co.uk. *Foods free of gluten, wheat and dairy.*
Green's 0113 250 2036; www.glutenfreebeers.co.uk. *Gluten/wheat-free beers.*
Gluten Free Foods 020 8953 4444; www.glutenfree-foods.co.uk. *Producers of the Glutano, Barkat, Tritamyl and Valpiform ranges.*

Heron Quality Foods +353 (0)23 39006; www.glutenfreedirect.com. *Irish co-operative producing wheat- and gluten-free foods.*

Matthew Foods 0800 028 4499; www.purespreads.com. *Dairy-free spreads.*

Meridian Foods 01490 413151; www.meridianfoods.co.uk. *Wheat- and dairy-free sauces, spreads and condiments.*

Nutricia 01225 711801; www.glutafin.co.uk. *Makers of Glutafin gluten-free range.*

Orgran 020 8208 2966; www.orgran.com. *A selection of snacks, cereals and pastas free of gluten, wheat, dairy and egg.*

Plamil Foods 01303 854207; www.plamilfoods.co.uk. *Non-dairy milks, chocolate and drinks, and egg-free mayonnaises.*

Provamel 0800 018 8180; www.provamel.co.uk. *Makers of Alpro, soya-based milks, creams, yogurts and desserts.*

Soma Organics 0870 950 7662; www.somafoods.com. *Producers of the nightshade-free Nomato range of baked beans, ketchup, soup, chilli and pasta sauce.*

Tofutti 020 8861 4443; www.tofutti.co.uk. *Dairy-free desserts.*

Trufree 01225 711801; www.trufree.co.uk. *Gluten and wheat-free bread, biscuits and pasta.*

The Village Baker 01768 881811; www.village-bakery.com. *Gluten, wheat and dairy-free cakes, puddings and fruit bars.*

Other

Dietarycard.co.uk. 01506 635358; www.dietarycard.co.uk. *Personalised food alert cards for use in hotels and restaurants in the UK and abroad, with translations available in several European languages to help articulate specific intolerances and dietary needs.*

Further reading

Bear in mind when consulting related literature that variant definitions of both food intolerance and food allergy may have been used.

Books and publications

Brewer, Dr Sarah, and Berriedale-Johnson, Michelle, *The IBS Diet*, Thorsons, 2004

Brody, Karen, *Coping with Coeliac Disease*, Sheldon Press, 1997

Brostoff, Professor Jonathan, and Gamlin, Linda, *The Complete Guide to Food Allergy and Intolerance*, Bloomsbury, 1998

Committee on Toxicity of Chemicals in Food, Consumer Products and the Environment, *Adverse Reactions to Food and Food Ingredients*, FSA, 2000

Emsley, John, and Fell, Peter, *Was it Something You Ate?*, OUP, 1999

Hanssen, Maurice, and Marsden, Jill, *New E for Additives*, Harper-Collins, 1987

Lipski, Elizabeth, *Digestive Wellness*, Keats, 1996

Orbach, Susie, *On Eating*, Penguin, 2002

Marsden, Kathryn, *Good Gut Healing*, Piatkus, 2003

Royal College of Physicians, *Allergy: the Unmet Need*, RCP, 2003

Savill, Antoinette, *The Big Book of Wheat-free Cooking*, Thorsons, 2004

Scott-Moncrieff, Christina, *Overcoming Allergies*, Collins and Brown, 2002

Ursell, Amanda, *L is for Labels*, Hay House, 2004

Magazines

Allergy Magazine
Ink, 141–143 Shoreditch High Street, London E1 6JE
Tel: 020 7613 8777
Email: allergy@electricink.com
Website: www.allergymagazine.com

Foods Matter Magazine
5 Lawn Road, London NW3 2XS
Tel: 020 7722 2866
Email: info@foodsmatter.com
Website: www.foodsmatter.com

Living Without Magazine
P.O. Box 2126
Northbrook, IL 60065, USA
Tel: 00 1 (847) 480 8810
Email: editor@LivingWithout.com
Website: www.LivingWithout.com

Index

n.b. Please refer to Chapter 3 for specific symptoms and complaints, listed alphabetically (abdominal pain, arthritis, asthma etc.)